CW01272702

Nature's Morphology
An Atlas of Tooth Shape and Form

NATURE'S MORPHOLOGY

An Atlas of Tooth Shape and Form

Shigeo Kataoka, RDT
Osaka, Japan

Yoshimi Nishimura, RDT
Osaka, Japan

Avishai Sadan, DMD
Editor of the English Edition
Louisiana State University
New Orleans, Louisiana

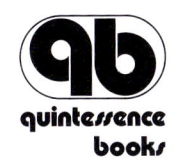

Quintessence Publishing Co, Inc

Chicago, Berlin, Tokyo, Copenhagen, London, Paris, Milan, Barcelona, Istanbul, São Paulo, New Delhi, Moscow, Prague, and Warsaw

Library of Congress Cataloging-in-Publication Data

Kataoka, Shigeo.
  Nature's morphology : an atlas of tooth shape and form / Shigeo Kataoka, Yoshimi Nishimura ; Avishai Sadan, editor of the English edition.
      p. ; cm.
   ISBN 0-86715-411-X (hardback)
1. Teeth—Anatomy—Atlases.
   [DNLM: 1. Dental Restoration, Permanent—methods—Atlases. 2. Esthetics, Dental—Atlases. 3. Tooth—anatomy & histology—Atlases. 4. Tooth—physiology—Atlases. WU 317 K19n 2002] I. Nishimura, Yoshimi. II. Sadan, Avishai. III. Title.
   QM311 .K34 2002
    611'.314—dc21

2002003732

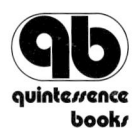

© 2002 Quintessence Publishing Co, Inc

Quintessence Publishing Co, Inc
551 Kimberly Drive
Carol Stream, Illinois 60188
www.quintpub.com

All rights reserved. This book or any part thereof may not be reproduced, stored in a retrieval system, or transmitted in any form or by any means, electronic, mechanical, photocopying, recording, or otherwise, without prior written permission of the publisher.

Editor: Arinne Dickson
Production: Susan Robinson

Printed in Japan

Dedication

This book is dedicated to the renowned master ceramist Makoto Yamamoto, a source of guidance and inspiration; and to the staff of Osaka Ceramic Training Center, for their dedication and support of this project.

Table of Contents

Preface to the English Edition 8
Avishai Sadan

Preface to the Japanese Edition 9
Shigeo Kataoka

Preface to the Japanese Edition 11
Yoshimi Nishimura

Chapter 1 Fundamentals of Tooth Morphology 13
  The Three Basic Shapes of Tooth Crown Morphology 14
  Transition of the Three Basic Morphologies Toward Successive Teeth 22

Chapter 2 Characteristics of Tooth Morphology 25
  Various Forms of Natural Teeth 26
  Three Typical Forms of Natural Teeth 28
  Characteristics of the Labial Surface 30
  Characteristics of the Lingual Surface 32
  Characteristics of the Proximal Surfaces 34
  Transition Between Surfaces 36
  Reproduction of the Form with Well-Developed Marginal Ridges 38
  Reproduction of the Basic Form 40
  Reproduction of the Form Without Particular Characteristics 42

Chapter 3 The Effect of Aging on Tooth Morphology 45
  Changes in Tooth Appearance 46
  Extrinsic Factors that Affect the Appearance of Tooth Crowns 48
  Expression of Changes in Tooth Morphology and Dentition with Age 50

Chapter 4 Contouring Ceramic Restorations I 55

    Contouring a Single Restoration 56
    Adjustment of Proximal Contact Areas 58
    Gross Contouring I: Three-Plane Labial Composition 60
    Gross Contouring II: Marginal Ridges and Proximal Transitional Surfaces 62
    Gross Contouring III: Lingual Surface 64
    Intermediate Finishing I: Line Angles, Transitional Areas, and Primary Ridges 66
    Intermediate Finishing II: Transverse Ridges and Grooves 68
    Finishing I: Gross Surface Texture 70
    Finishing II: Detailed Surface Texture and Polishing 72
    Completion 74
    Examples of Single Restorations 76

Chapter 5 Contouring Ceramic Restorations II 79

    Contouring a Three-Unit Fixed Partial Denture 80
    Gross Contouring I: Incisal Edge Length and Three-Plane Labial Composition 82
    Gross Contouring II: Midline Area (Interproximal Space) 84
    Gross Contouring III: Proximal Transitional Surfaces and Individualization 86
    Intermediate Finishing I: Proximal Transitional Surface 88
    Intermediate Finishing II: Labial Ridges 90
    Finishing I: Proximal Area and Lingual Grooves 92
    Finishing II: Surface Characterization and Polishing 94
    Completed Fixed Partial Denture 96

Preface to the English Edition

Many factors contribute to the successful fabrication of the inconspicuous esthetic restoration. However, the key factor that takes precedence over all other components is proper shape reproduction. It takes more than an ordinary knowledge of tooth morphology to achieve extraordinary results, and at this level no detail is too trivial.

Fixed prosthodontics is a clinical science stabilized on three legs of a tripod: the dentist, the dental technician, and the dental biomaterials researcher. Each of them contributes equally to our understanding of the clinical procedures, technical approaches, and material selection. Despite their importance, however, morphology stands alone. While most of the materials and clinical and technical procedures are judged within the context of time and continue to evolve, morphology is timeless and unchanging. A thorough understanding of morphology is a wealth one will cherish and use far beyond the boundaries of ever-changing techniques and materials. The increased popularity of direct and semidirect anterior restorations has made this book an indispensable source for dentists, though it was originally written for dental technicians.

Japan's finest ceramists have been respected for their unique ability to observe the smallest of details, to document them accurately, to distill them to a methodical concept that can be easily taught, and to have the incredible discipline to consistently reproduce those details. Mr Shigeo Kataoka and Mr Yoshimi Nishimura are the finest examples of this tradition. Not only are they world-renowned masters in their field, they are experienced teachers who have trained many generations of students; some of their students are renowned masters themselves.

The most demanding challenge Mr Kataoka and Mr Nishimura faced in presenting the topic of morphology was the need to isolate it from all other components of the dental restoration, such as shade and materials. While natural teeth, in situ or extracted, or artificial restorations could have been used to demonstrate their concepts, these approaches would still present many distractions, such as shade. Thus, they selected an approach that combines waxups, casts, and illustrations. Only at the end of each chapter are examples of dental restorations displayed.

I invite you to sit down and enjoy the book. It has multiple layers. As Mr Nishimura suggests, start by looking at the illustrations. Since the text is extremely technical at times, it may take a few readings to absorb it, but it will be time well spent. Any technician or dentist working on anterior teeth will greatly benefit from this book, and its timelessness will make it a useful reference for many years to come.

Avishai Sadan, DMD
Department of Prosthodontics
Louisiana State University School of Dentistry

Preface to the Japanese Edition

The magnificent image of trees reaching to the sky and fallen trees nearby still budding and not decaying was the inspiration for the title of this book, *Nature's Morphology*, since the same malleable beauty that nature creates in trees can be found in the human dentition. The morphology of the natural tooth is our ideal guide, and close observation of it will teach us about how it functions, about its relationship to the periodontal tissues, and about how it creates harmony with a person's face. With natural dentition as our model, this book provides instruction for attaining harmony in dental restorations.

The growing demand for esthetic restorations was a major impetus for the commercial development of ceramic materials with improved esthetic properties. As a result, modern ceramics enable the ceramist to attain a natural look in artificial restorations, which requires the successful reproduction of three critical aspects: single-tooth morphology, tooth alignment, and natural tooth color.

To create pleasing esthetics, these three elements must achieve a delicate balance. This book discusses reproduction of single-tooth morphology and tooth alignment in detail. As masters in this field know, reproduction of natural tooth color is closely related to morphology, although it is traditionally not considered to be. Various build-up techniques have been introduced, but their outcome is similar: a color composition of several layers of porcelain. The proper expression of color is the result of properly layering the different colors within the overall space confinements available for the porcelain. In other words, the harmony of the esthetic restoration is a balance of color and proper morphology. One can achieve this goal only with a thorough understanding and expert reproduction of morphology.

Morphology is the foundation of dental laboratory work; therefore, understanding the proper technique for its reproduction is paramount. This is the main reason why morphology is the topic of this book.

Three fundamental elements of morphology are necessary to create esthetically pleasing restorations:

1. The first is knowledge of the three basic tooth morphologies—square, ovoid, and tapered—and the ability to adapt each to harmonize with the patient's face and dentition.
2. The second is a mastery of lobes, which are the elements that compose morphology. Lobes are considered anatomic divisions of a tooth and are usually separated by primary grooves. All human teeth comprise four or more lobes. Because tooth surfaces are interrelated and do not exist as separate entities, a complete understanding of lobes is essential to creating the proper composition of a tooth. The connections between the various surfaces form the tooth. Therefore, one must know how to relate surfaces to each other to achieve an esthetic contour of the crown. The degree to which each lobe is developed will dictate its relationship with the next lobe, and thus will dictate the direction, thickness, and location of connection between the lobes. This will also determine location, distinctiveness, and depth of grooves and pits. It is easy to see that tooth morphology is the sum of the various lobes and their interaction.

3. Surface texture is the third factor that determines the esthetic outcome of the ceramic crown. The knowledge of surface texture and ability to create it enables us to express processes such as aging. This may be one of the most difficult techniques to teach.

Since nature is the only model for our work, thorough observation and accumulation of knowledge of natural teeth, in conjunction with practice and experience, are key to developing the proper skills for the fabrication of a dental restoration.

This book is written with the hope that young technicians will create their own bright future by striving to understand the proper morphology of a single tooth.

I would like to thank the staff of Osaka Ceramic Training Center and Kataoka Ceramic. I am especially grateful to Mr Yuji Okubo and Mr Tayu Wakita, who created the illustrations for this book. It is difficult to find the proper words to express my deepest appreciation to Mr Makoto Yamamoto, who dedicated many hours to guide us at every stage of preparation for this book, from photography and manuscript writing to page layout and proofing. His support was paramount.

Shigeo Kataoka, RDT
Director, Osaka Ceramic Training Center

Preface to the Japanese Edition

Only a thorough understanding of dental anatomy can result in the proper expression of tooth morphology in dental restorations. Although I had studied dental anatomy during my training, and many excellent textbooks on dental anatomy were available to me, I paid little attention to these sources until about 10 years ago.

Why did I not pay attention to these books? It seems to me that none was written by people who actually fabricate dental restorations—dental technicians—and therefore the books were unappealing to me.

After realizing this, I contemplated the feasibility of putting together a book that would describe dental anatomy from a technician's point of view. Fortunately, an invitation to write such a book came from a publisher and thus enabled us to crystalize our thoughts.

Regardless of future advancements in dentistry, either from a biologic or biomaterials standpoint, the concept of reproducing natural tooth morphology in dental restorations remains timeless. In addition, creating harmony with the periodontal apparatus and jaw movements and providing durability are some other crucial factors that one should address when fabricating dental restorations.

We initially envisioned a textbook that could be understood simply by studying illustrations. However, as the work progressed, we found it impossible to convey all of our thoughts without text. The text in this book, as in dental anatomy books, is full of technical terms and attempts to explain three-dimensional objects. Trying to absorb all of the information from the images and text in the first reading is an unnecessary challenge. I suggest that you start by looking at the images first, then read the text.

Working on this book made me realize how quickly time passes and how much effort is required to generate such a publication. Writing a book while holding a full-time position is no easy task and would have been impossible without the tremendous support of many people. With Mr Kataoka, I extend heartfelt gratitude to Mr Makoto Yamamoto. His advice about book preparation was indispensable. I also thank the staff at Dental Creation Art for their faithful support during this project, and the staff at Osaka Ceramic Training Center and M. Yamamoto Ceramist's, Inc, knowing that we significantly inconvenienced them during the preparation of this book.

Yoshimi Nishimura, RDT
Dental Creation Art

CHAPTER 1

Fundamentals of Tooth Morphology

The Three Basic Shapes of Tooth Crown Morphology

Besides the fundamental requirements of proper fit and occlusion, an important criterion for the success of a ceramic crown is its ability to integrate and exist in harmony within the intraoral and extraoral environments. The ability to establish this harmony is the most important factor in judging the success of a restoration. When forming a restoration, one carefully studies and evaluates many factors, such as tooth alignment, clinical crown size, occlusion, and the like, because the proper understanding and reproduction of these factors will create a harmonious restoration. Therefore, this book will emphasize the morphology of the clinical crown.

Facial shapes as well as tooth shapes exist in different forms. As the shapes of faces are different from each other, so is the morphology of teeth. In 1912 J.L. William et al theorized that for each person a certain relationship exists between the shape of the face and the shape of the teeth. Some still consider this theory valid for the formation of anterior tooth restoration, though this concept is rarely applied to clinical use. However, the Bioblend porcelain tooth selection method by Dentsply is an exception. This method is based on selecting a tooth shape similar to the facial shape and uses four basic facial shapes: square, square-tapered, tapered, and ovoid. The shape of the face is noted, the width and length of the face are measured, and one sixteenth of each measurement is calculated. With these measurements, the six maxillary anterior teeth that belong to that facial shape are selected.

The J.L. William concept is used in removable prosthodontics but not in fixed prosthodontics in part because a clinical manual for the fabrication of fixed partial dentures based on facial shape does not exist. Without such guidelines, the experienced technician tends to fabricate a restoration with morphology that reflects personal preference, and the inexperienced technician may encounter difficulties selecting and designing the proper shape of a restoration. Needless to say, the field of fixed prosthodontics has long needed such a manual.

This chapter analyzes and discusses a concept that is based on three basic shapes of a tooth crown. Using the maxillary central incisor as a model, the chapter addresses all tooth surfaces. This concept of three basic crown shapes is also applicable to the lateral incisor and the canine. Porcelain-fused-to-metal restorations that are fabricated according to this concept are presented at the end of the chapter.

ch 1 | 15

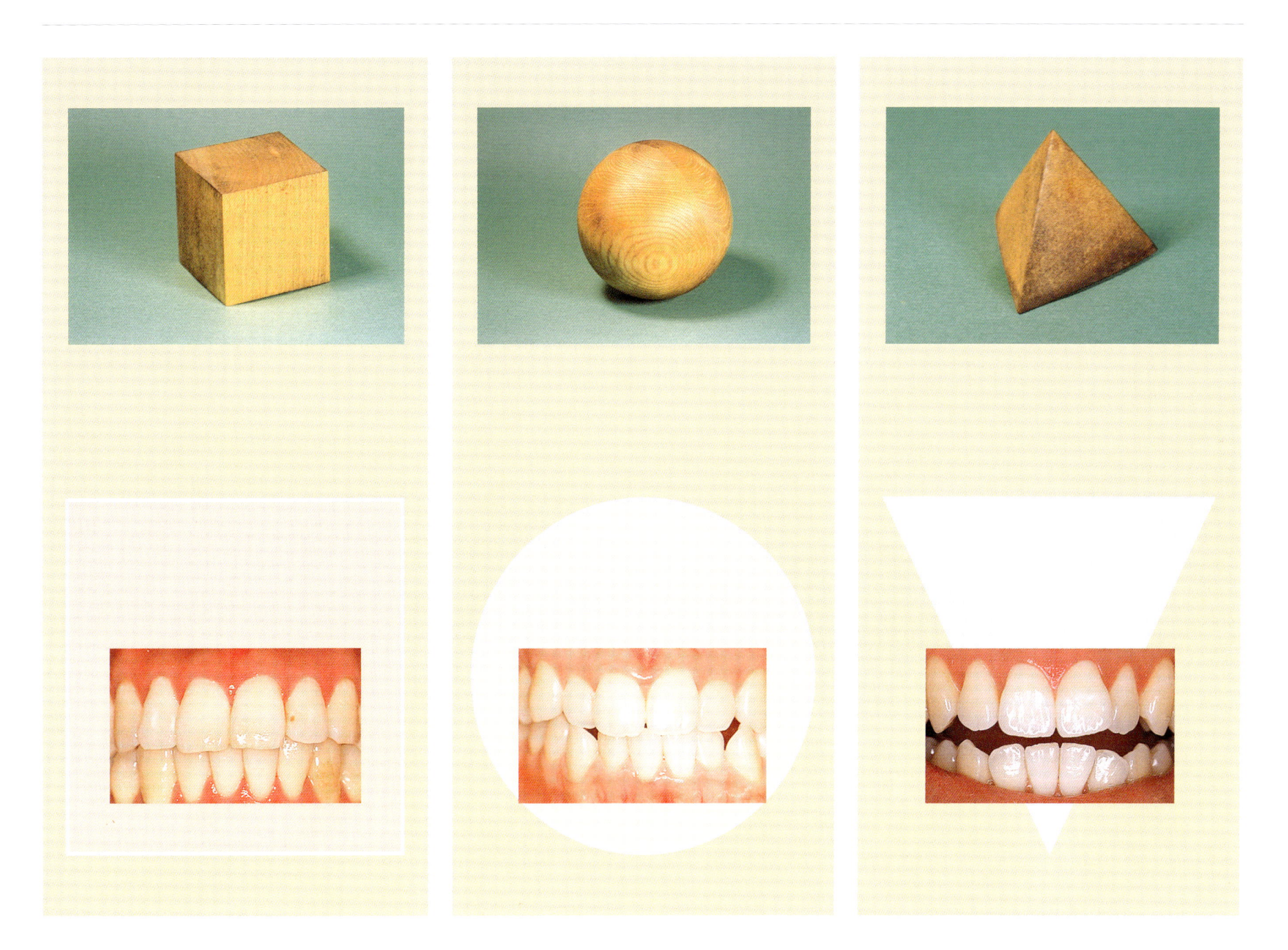

The Three Basic Shapes of Tooth Crown Morphology
Square

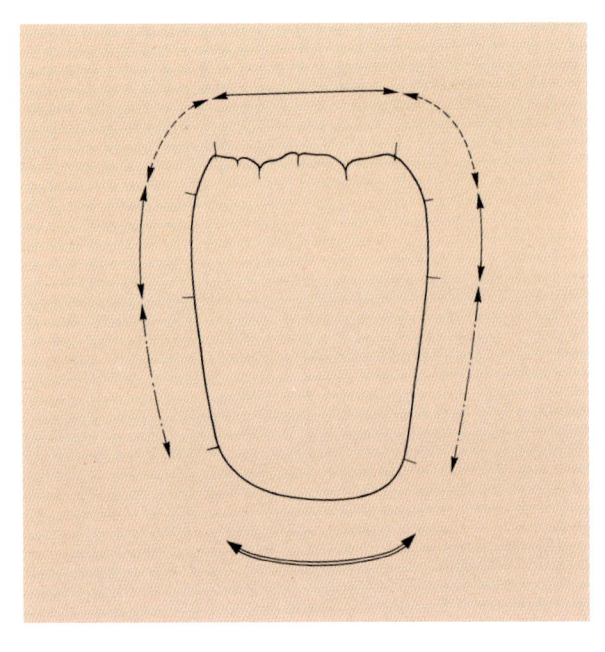

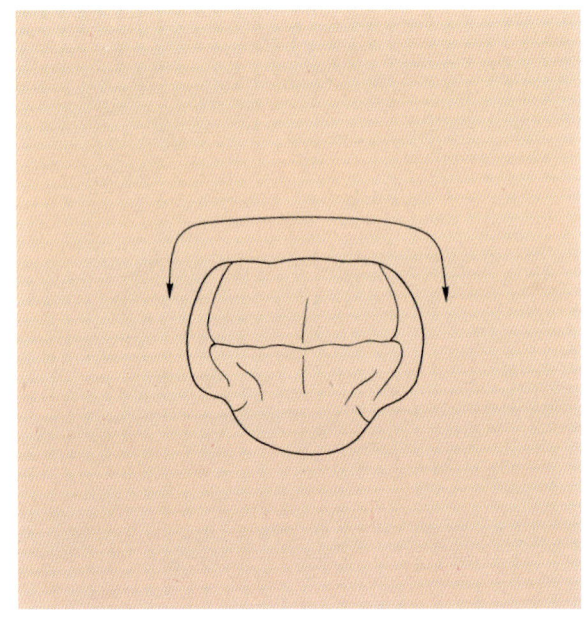

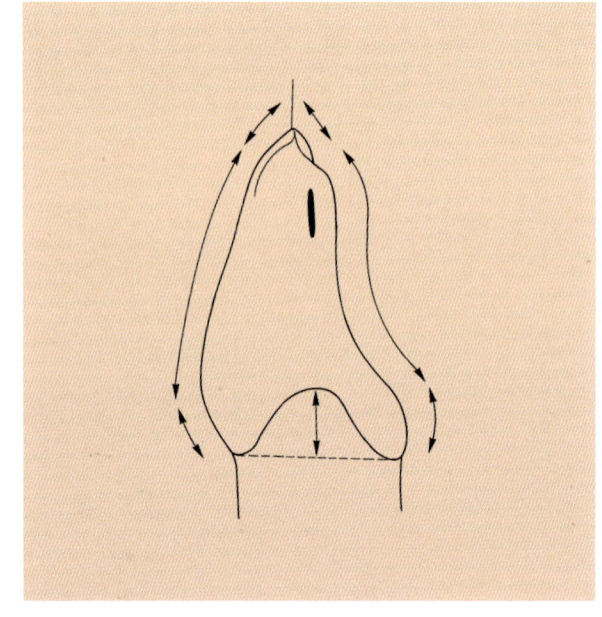

Labial view

- Incisal outline
  - Straight.
  - Mesiodistal length of the incisal edge is longer than that of the ovoid shape and about the same as the tapered shape.
- Incisal angles
  - The mesioincisal and distoincisal angles each approximate a right angle.
- Proximal outline
  - The mesial and distal proximal surfaces are parallel to each other and perpendicular to the incisal edge.
  - Slightly curved.
- Cervical line
  - A shallow U shape.
- Proximal contact areas
  - Long contact surface axially (incisogingivally). It is the longest contact surface of the three basic morphologies.

Incisal view

- Curvature of the tooth (horizontal plane of the incisal one third is visible)
  - Both marginal ridges are perpendicular to the incisal edge.
  - The incisal edge is straight mesiodistally.
  - It is the widest in the mesiodistal dimension among the three morphologies.
- Incisal point angles at the labial aspect
  - Mesiolabioincisal and distolabioincisal point angles approximate a right angle.
- Proximal outline
  - Proximal outlines are parallel to each other and perpendicular to the labial surface.
  - Straight with some convexity.

Proximal view

- Three labial planes
  - Middle plane is straight and long.
- Cervical line (coronal curvature)
  - It presents the least prominent curvature of the three basic morphologies.
- Depth of the cervical line curvature (the distance between the imaginary line connecting the lowest labiocervical point to the lowest linguocervical point [dotted line] to the highest point on the proximocervical line)
  - The proximal depth of the cervical line curvature is the shortest among the three morphologies.

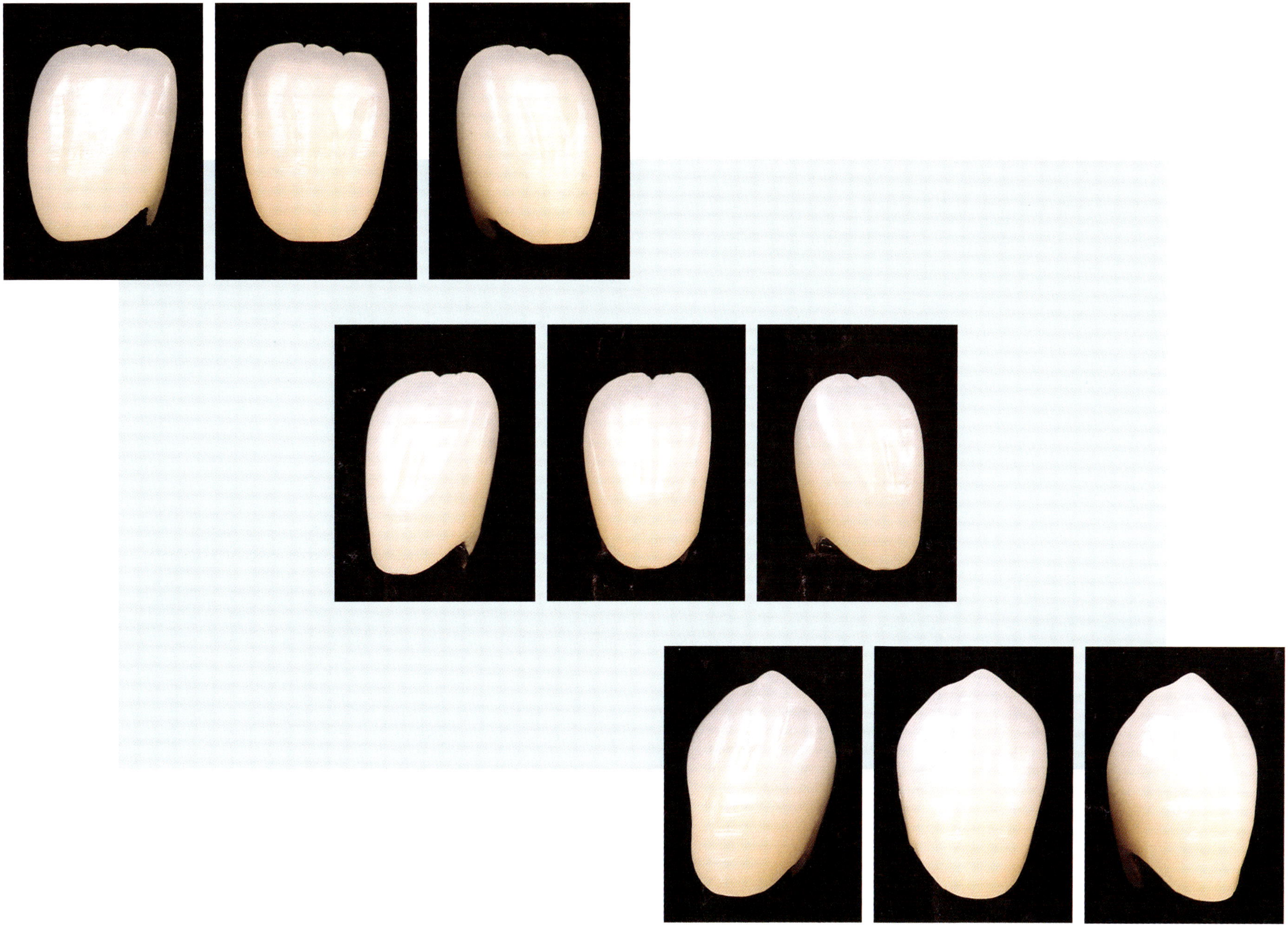

The Three Basic Shapes of Tooth Crown Morphology
Ovoid

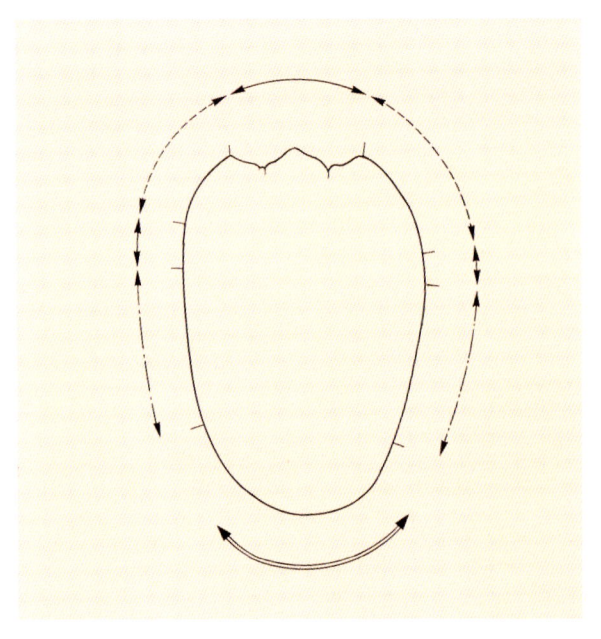

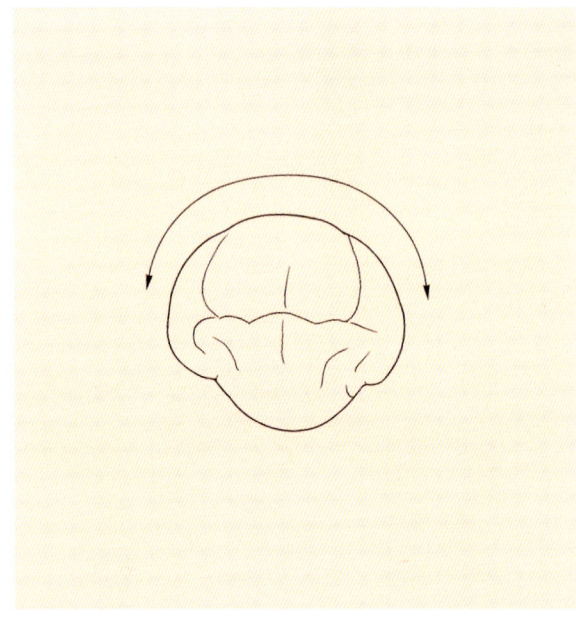

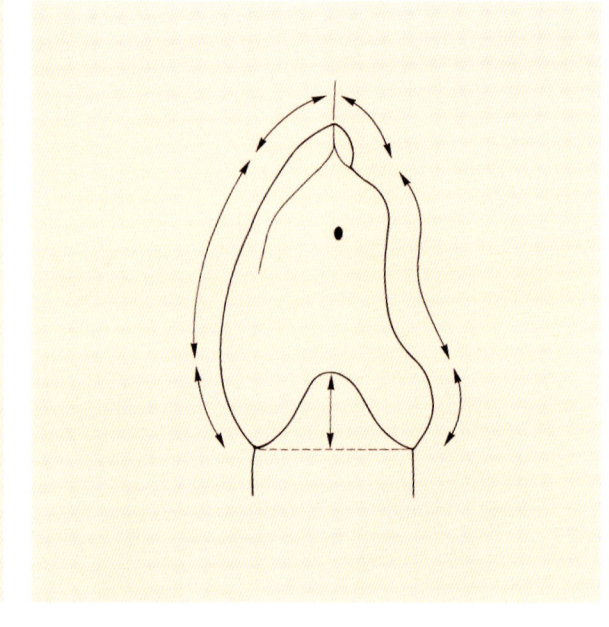

Labial view

- Incisal outline
  - It is elevated in the middle (convex).
  - Mesiodistal length of the incisal edge is the shortest of the three morphologies.
- Incisal angles
  - They are the most ovoid of the three morphologies.
- Proximal outline
  - The outline is narrower cervically than the square type.
  - Straight.
- Cervical line
  - The line is U-shaped and more ovoid than the square type.
- Proximal contact areas
  - They are in the middle of the proximal outline.
  - They are contact points rather than contact areas.

Incisal view

- Curvature of the tooth (horizontal plane of the incisal one third is visible)
  - The labial aspect is highly convex, and both lingual marginal ridges converge toward the lingual.
- Labial outline
  - The outline is ovoid in shape with convexity in the middle.
  - It is the narrowest mesiodistally among the three basic morphologies.
- Incisal point angles at the labial aspect
  - They are rounded with no definite corners.
- Proximal outline
  - The outline is convex mesiodistally and narrow lingually.
  - It shows rounded curvature.

Proximal view

- Three labial planes
  - Middle plane is rounded and relatively short.
- Cervical line
  - It shows moderately rounded curvature.
- Depth of the cervical line curvature
  - This depth is between the square and the tapered types.

ch 1 | 19

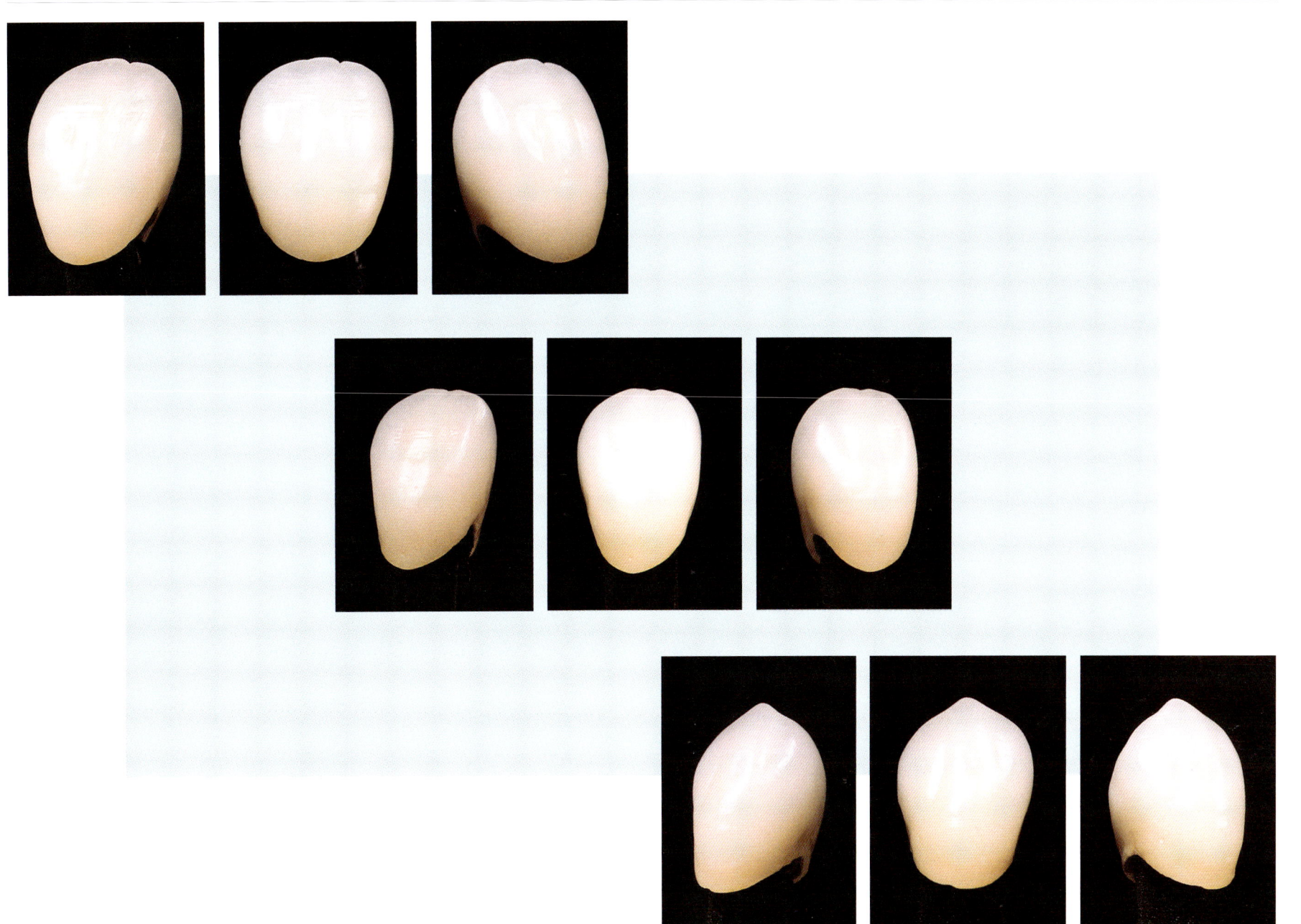

The Three Basic Shapes of Tooth Crown Morphology

Tapered

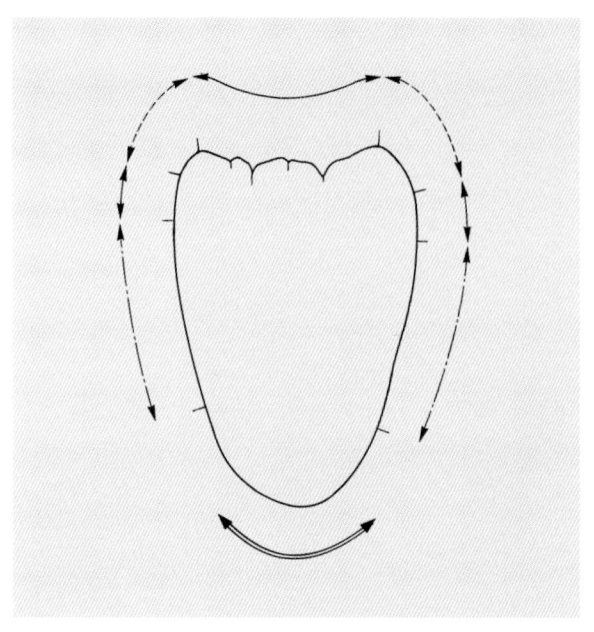

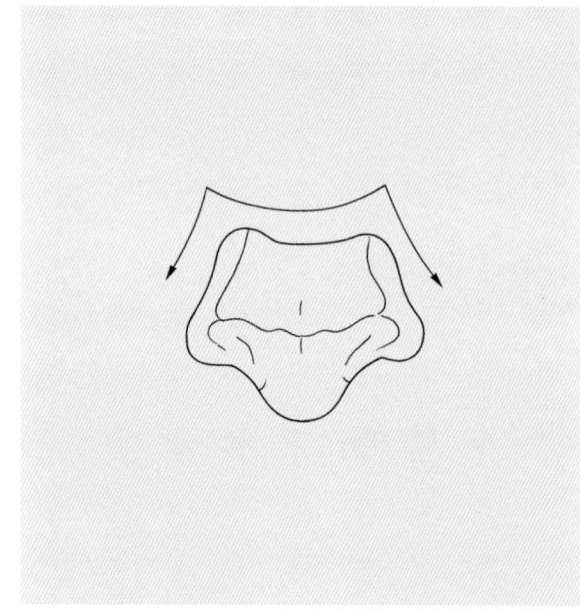

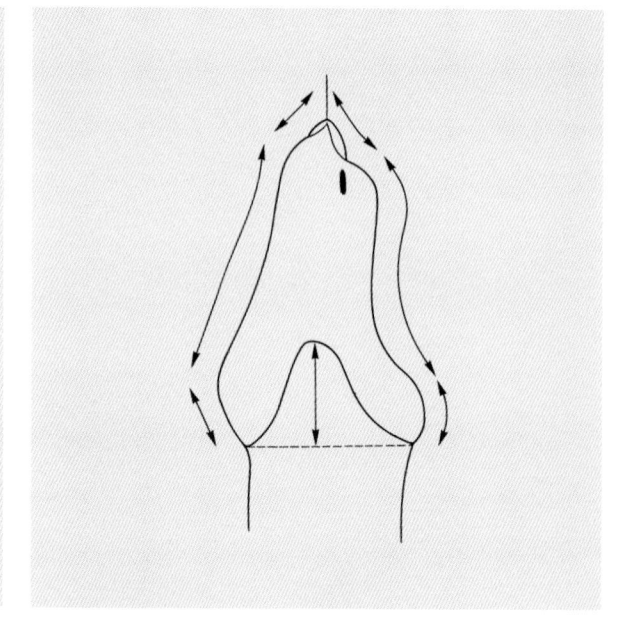

Labial view

- Incisal outline
  - It is concave in the middle.
  - Mesiodistal length of the incisal edge is longer than that of the ovoid shape and about the same as the square shape.
- Incisal angles
  - They are the sharpest of the three morphologies.
- Proximal outline
  - The outline is narrow cervically.
  - It is also straight.
- Cervical line
  - The line is V-shaped with the convexity in the middle of the crown.
- Proximal contact areas
  - The contact areas are near the incisal edge within the proximal outline.
  - Proximal contact areas are narrow.

Incisal view

- Curvature of the tooth (horizontal plane of the incisal one third is visible)
  - The curvature is concave on the labial side, and both lingual marginal ridges diverge from the lingual.
- Labial outline
  - Middle part is concave, and the mesial and distal ridges are prominent.
  - The width of the labial surface is between the square and the ovoid types.
- Incisal point angles at the labial aspect
  - They are rather obtuse angles.
- Proximal outline
  - The outline diverges lingually.
  - It is also straight.

Proximal view

- Three labial planes
  - Middle plane is concave. It is not visible, due to the mesial and distal marginal ridges.
- Cervical line
  - It is very prominently curved with a straight, sharp, reversed V-shape.
- Depth of the cervical line curvature
  - The proximal depth of the cervical line curvature is the deepest of the three morphologies.

ch 1 | 21

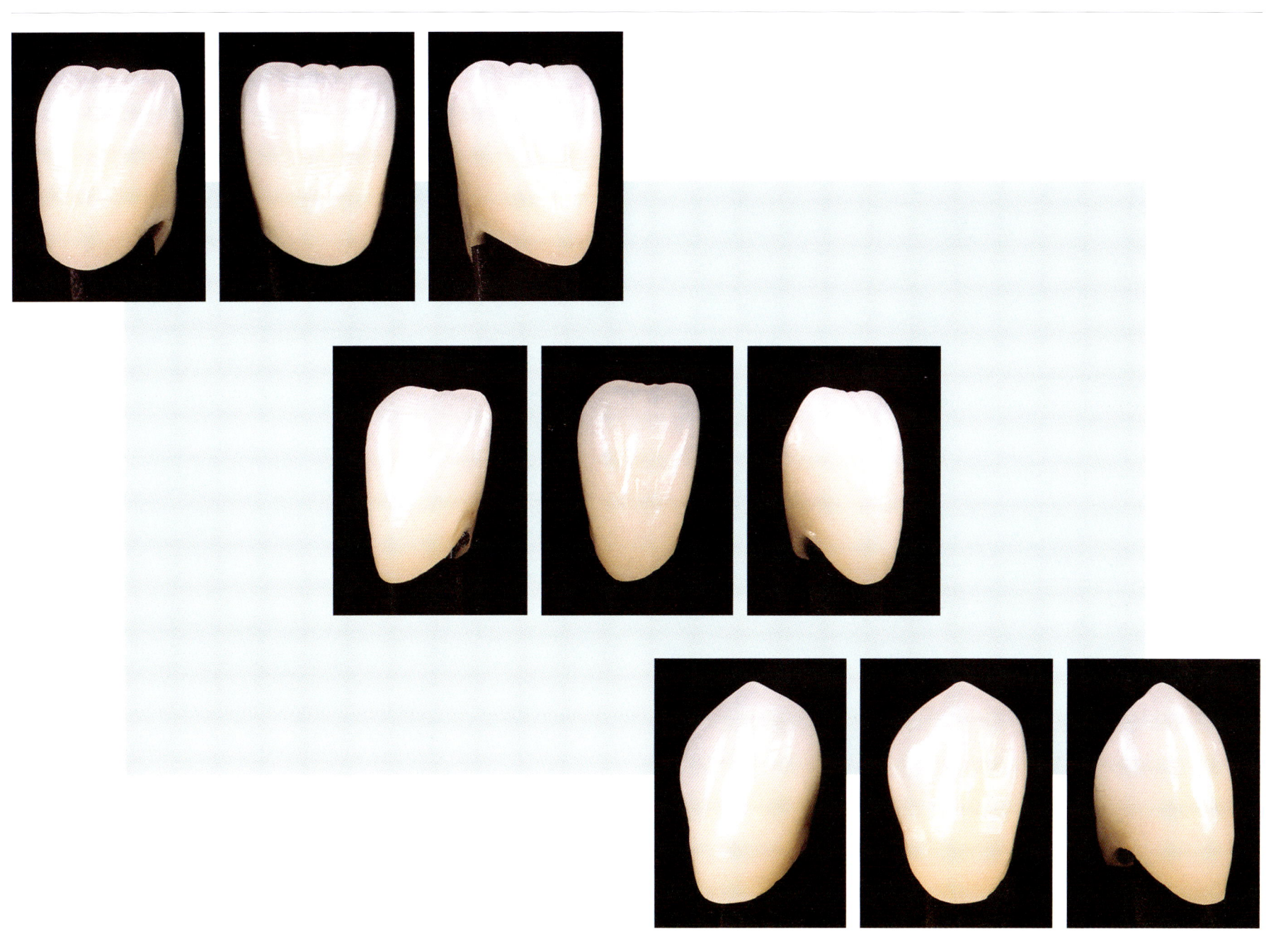

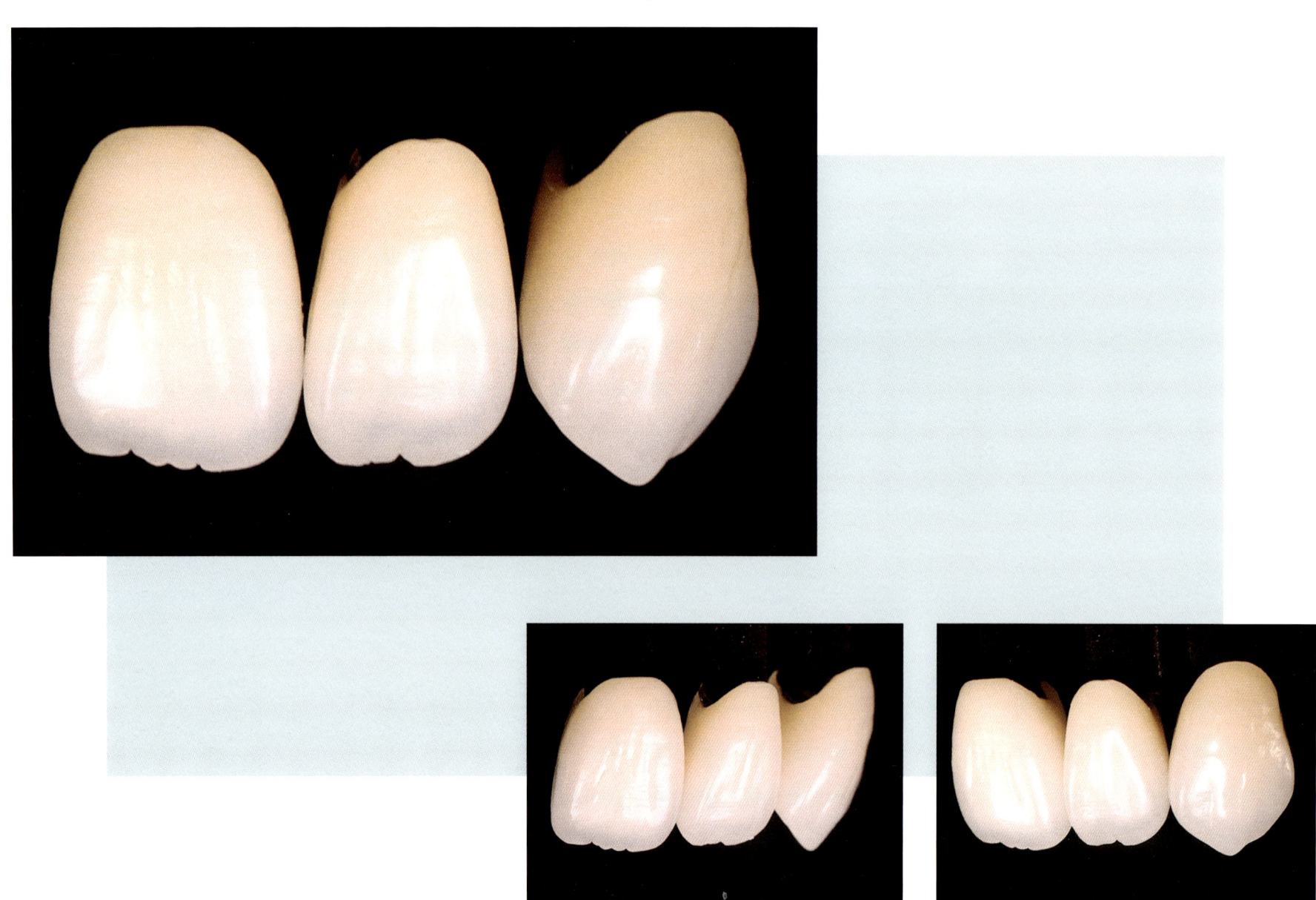

Transition of the Three Basic Morphologies Toward Successive Teeth
Square

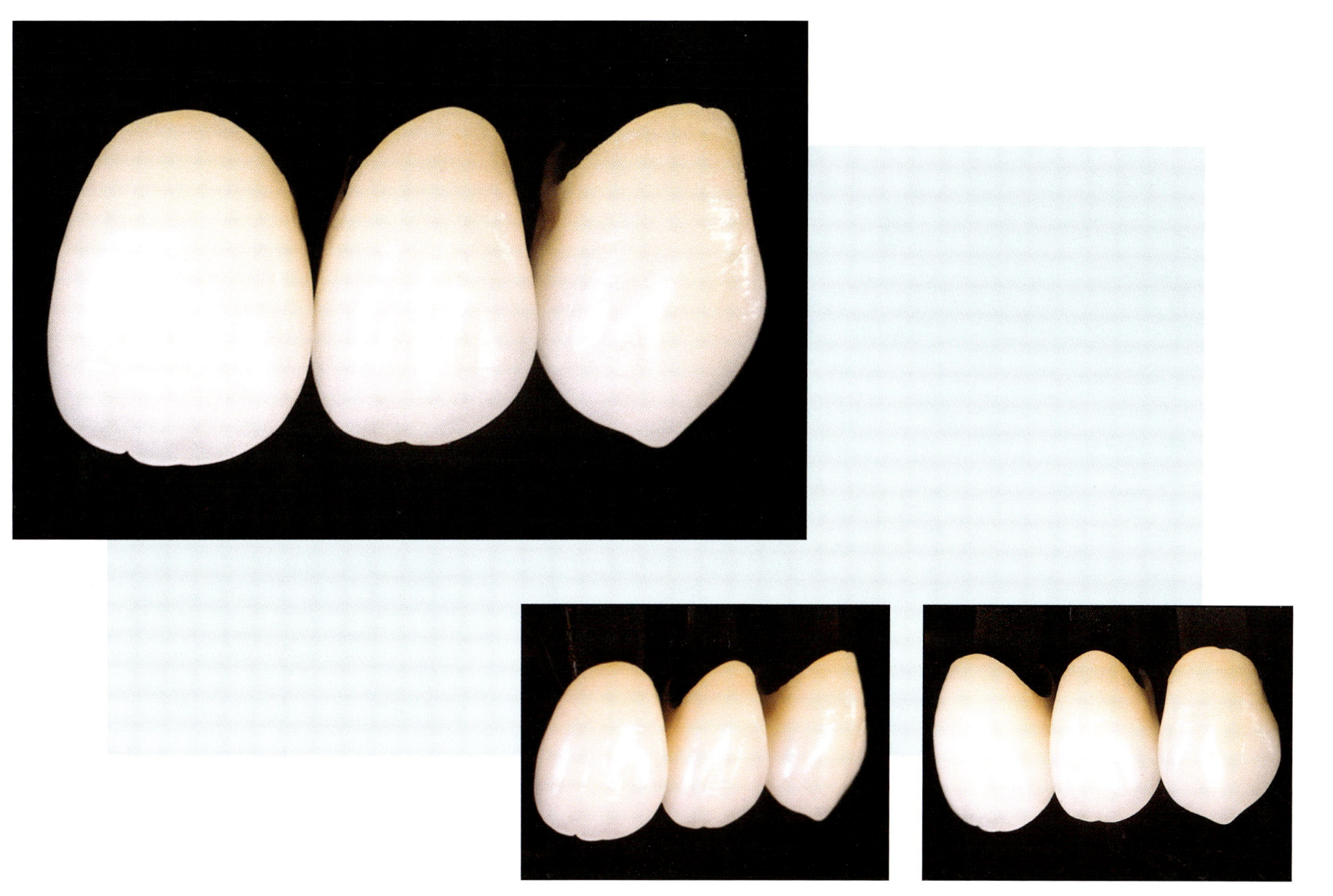

Ovoid

Transition of the Three Basic Morphologies Toward Successive Teeth
Tapered

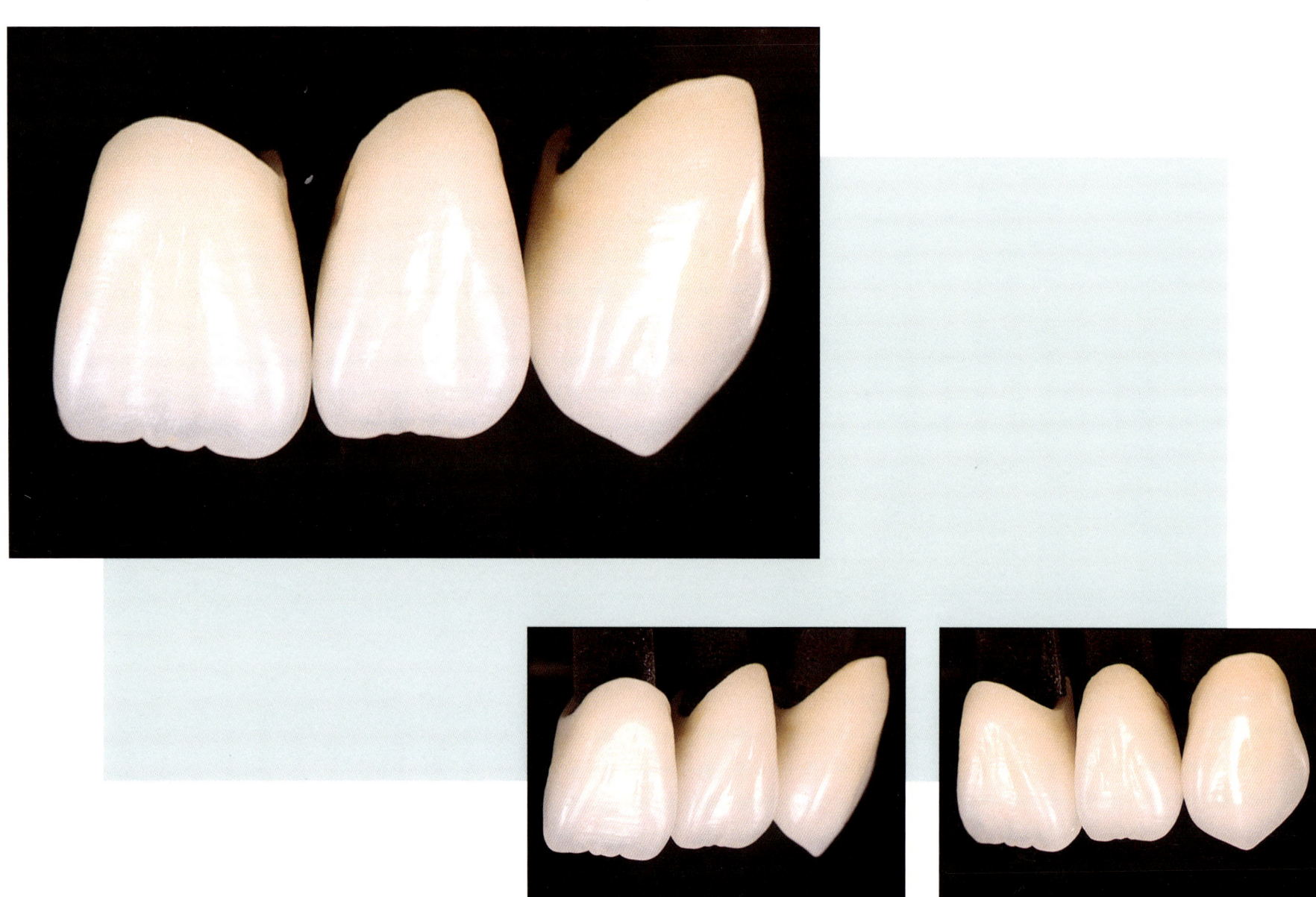

CHAPTER 2

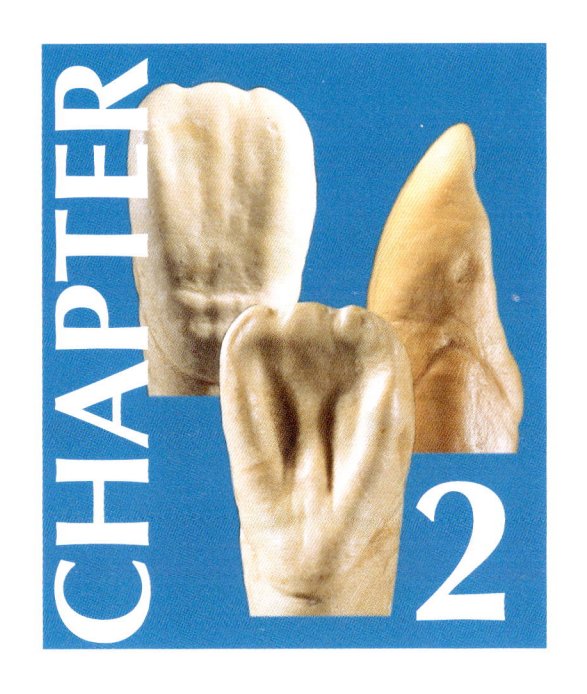

Characteristics of Tooth Morphology

Various Forms of Natural Teeth

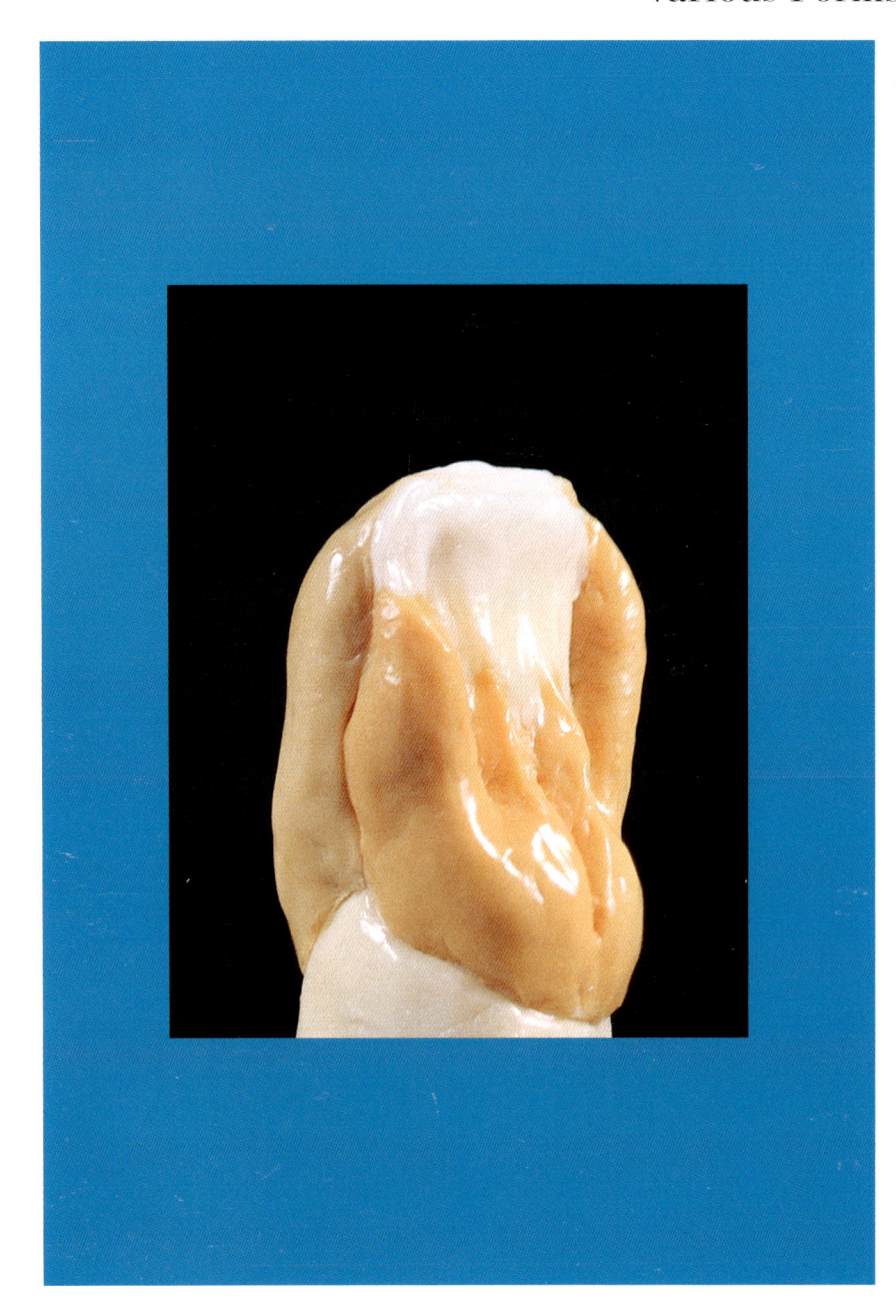

In the three types of tooth shape one can find many variations. These variations exist not only in the basic shape but also in tooth form. The term *form* in this context refers to gross characteristics, such as ridge development, groove depth, and differences between mesial and distal incisal corners, rather than to microcharacteristics, such as surface texture. To discuss the various characteristics of tooth form, this chapter identifies three typical forms.

Embryologically, a natural tooth is an assembly of elevations. When connected, these elevations form ridges. A good analogy for these connected elevations is mountains. Mountains have ridges and slopes that form valleys. The labial or lingual grooves in a natural tooth are analogous to mountain valleys.

While shaping a ceramic restoration, one should emphasize precise ridge formation and not focus on the formation of grooves and fossae. Since ridge formation also forms grooves and fossae, proper ridge reproduction will achieve them.

The pictures on this page and the opposing page demonstrate this concept well. The ridges, formed with clay over the white background, form the tooth shape as a whole, and the grooves and the fossae are formed as a result of ridge formation.

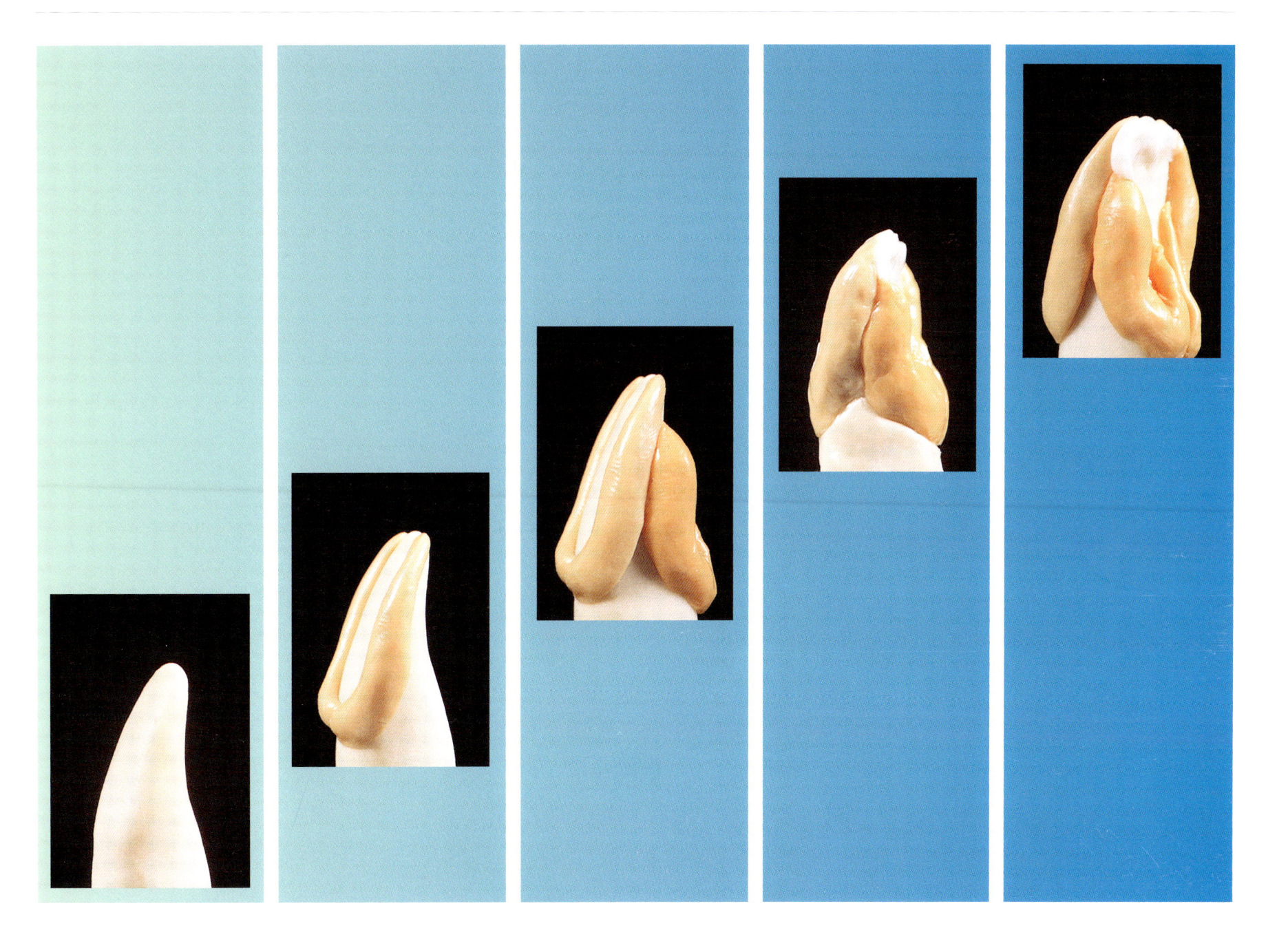

ch 2 | 27

Three Typical Forms of Natural Teeth

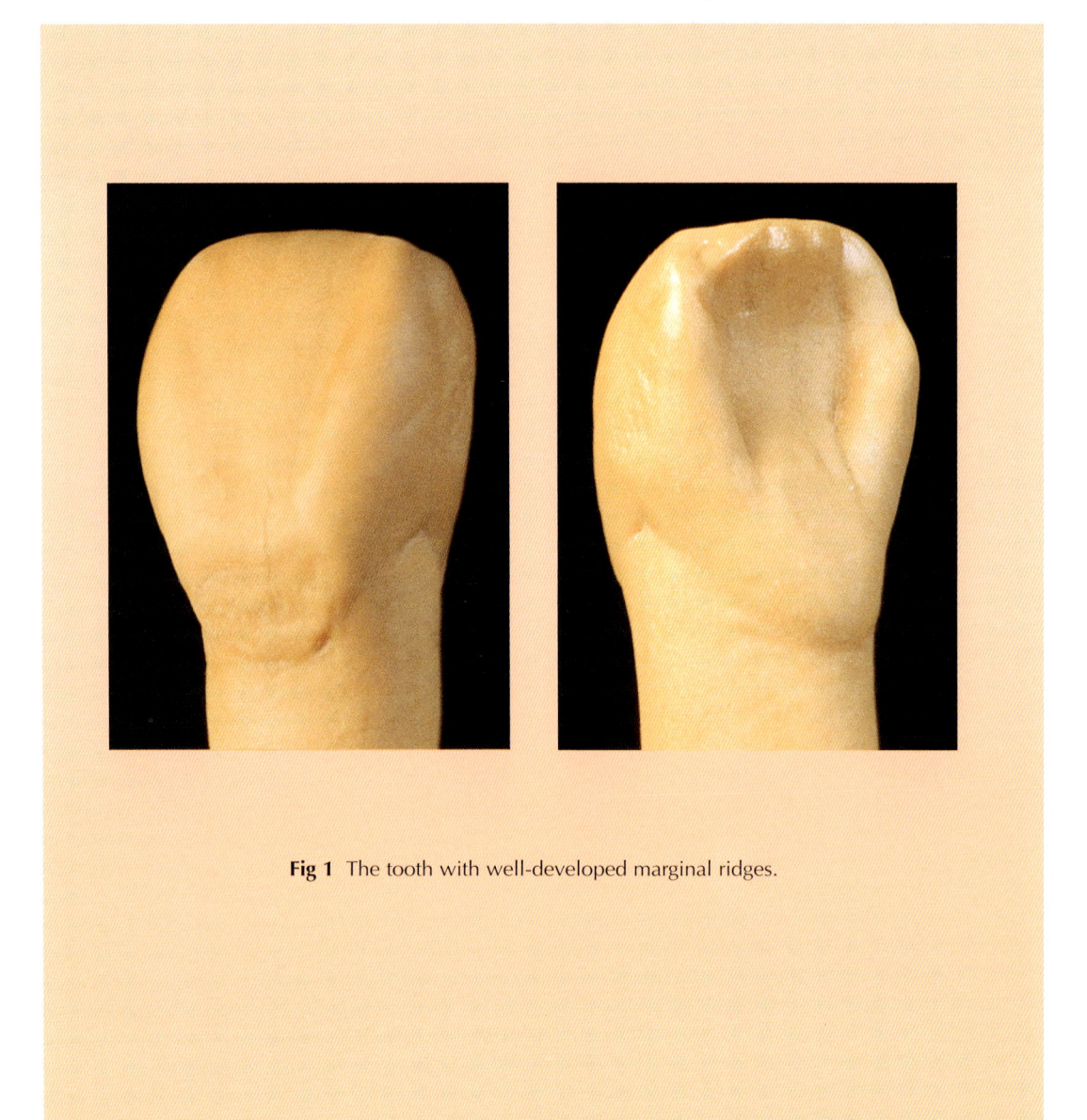

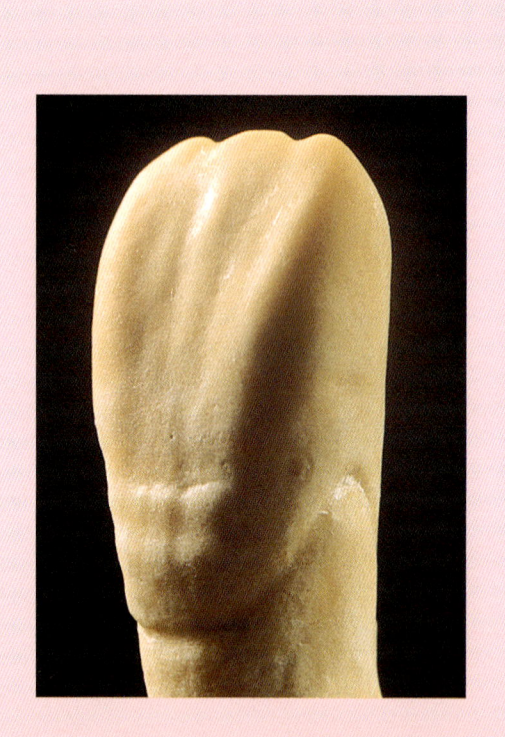

Fig 1 The tooth with well-developed marginal ridges.

Fig 2 The tooth with a basic form.

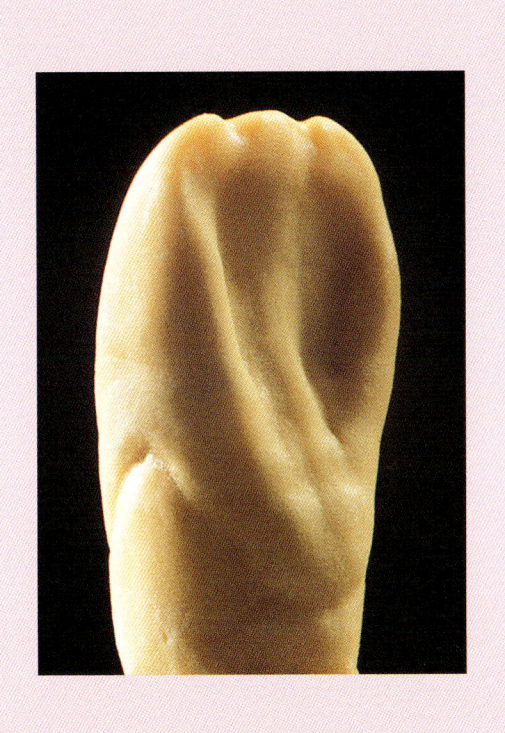

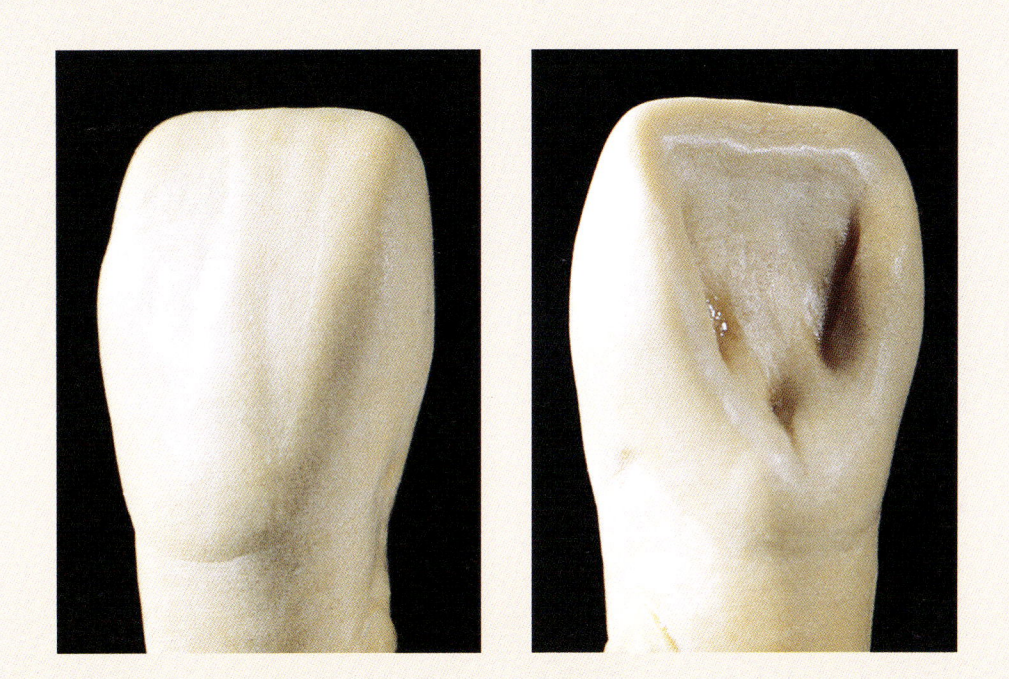

Fig 3 The tooth without particular characteristics.

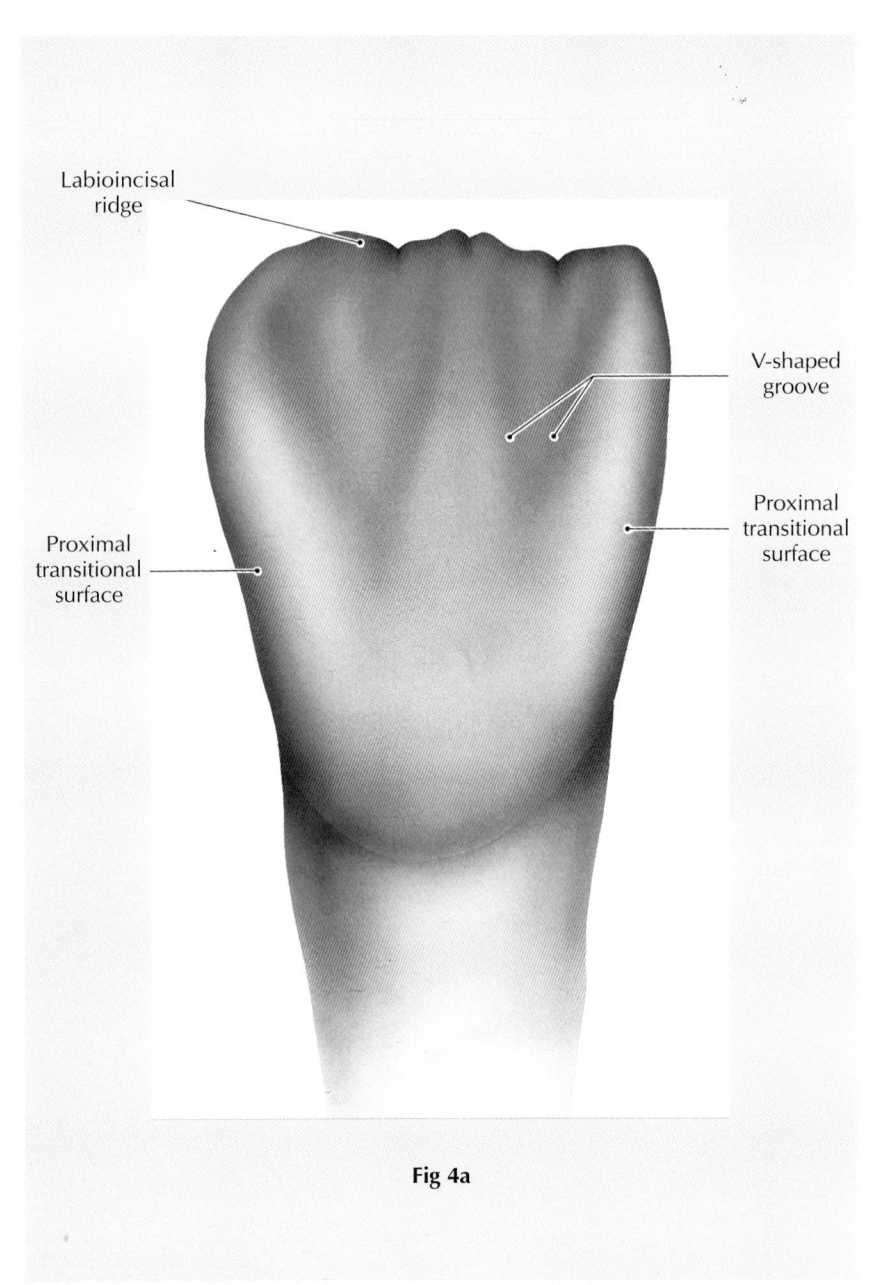

Characteristics of the Labial Surface

Fig 4a (labels: Labioincisal ridge; V-shaped groove; Proximal transitional surface; Proximal transitional surface)

Fig 4b (labels: Inner slope of the marginal ridge; Proximal transitional surface; Proximal groove; Incisal ridge; Twist of the labial surface)

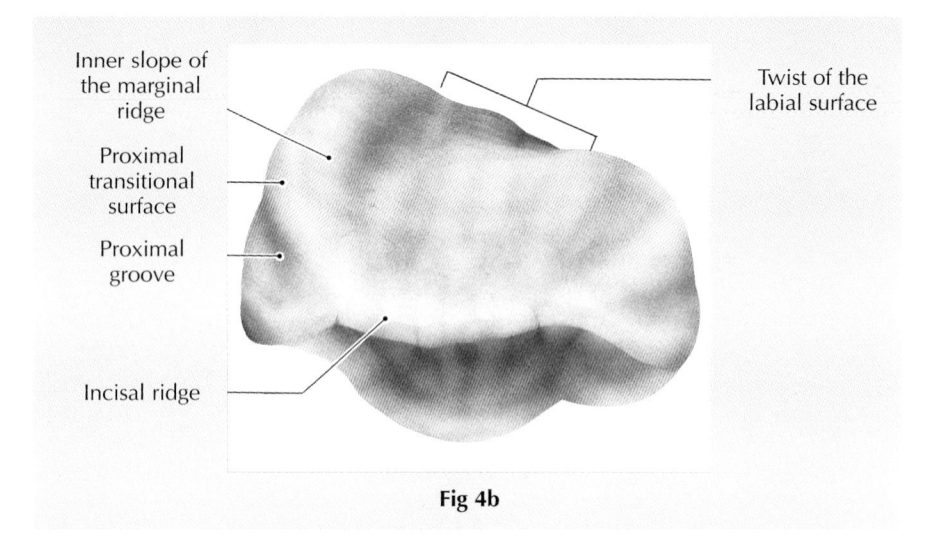

A central ridge runs through the middle of the labial surface from the incisal area cervically, and it forms slopes mesially and distally. There are marginal ridges on the mesiolabial and distolabial surfaces, which also form slopes mesially and distally. The inner slope of each marginal ridge and the slopes of the central ridge will form depressions between them; these are the labial grooves (also called the *labial developmental depressions*). The outer slope of each marginal ridge forms a convex surface, which is the transition to the proximal area; in this book these surfaces are called *proximal transitional surfaces*. The marginal ridges run from the incisal area toward the cervical area and form the mesial and distal outlines of the tooth crown. The outline of the incisal edge is formed by the incisal ridge from the lingual aspect, and the outline of the cervical area is formed by an enamel elevation at the cervical line (cementoenamel junction) that extends toward the coronal aspect. All of these ridges together create the outer form of the labial surface of the tooth crown.

Accessory ridges in the labial grooves form the V-shaped grooves, and transverse ridges are formed in the cervical area.

Fig 4c

Fig 4d

Fig 4e

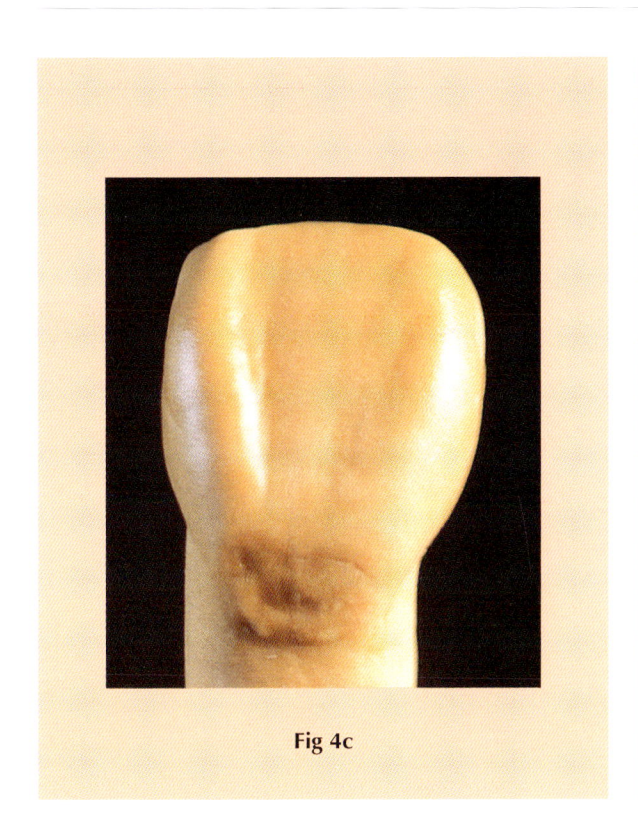

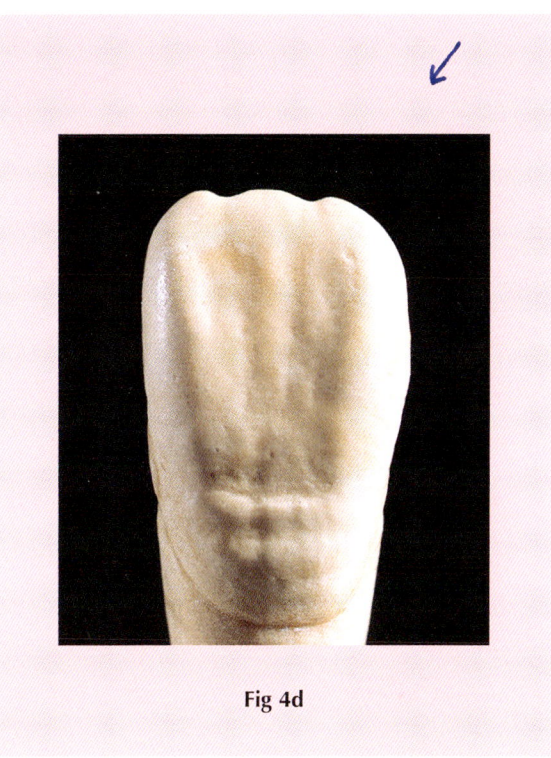

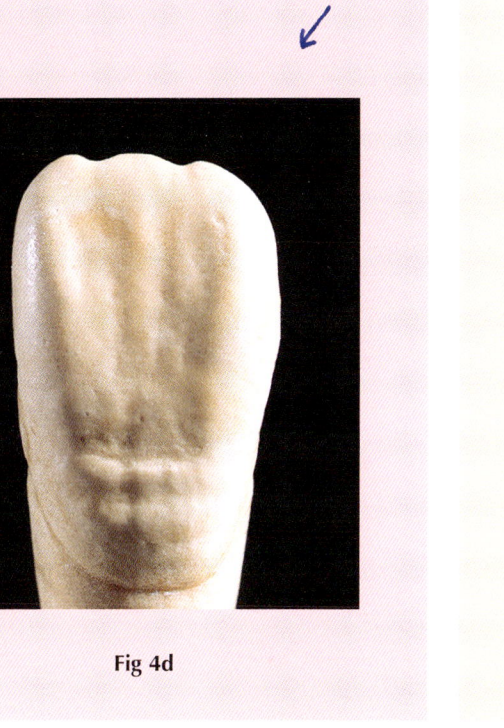

Labial surface analysis of the tooth form in Fig 1
The identifying characteristics of the labial surface of this tooth form are the well-developed marginal ridges. Teeth with this form present deep labial grooves and wide proximal transitional surfaces. The difference between the size of the mesial and distal proximal transitional surfaces is remarkable: the distal surface is wider than the mesial. In general, the lingual marginal ridges are well developed. The mesioincisal and distoincisal line angles have different shapes. The mesioincisal line angle is angled, and the distoincisal line angle is rounded. Furthermore, the labial accessory ridges and the V-shaped grooves are not well developed, and the labial surface appears concave and twisted from an incisal view. In general, the transverse grooves and ridges are not well formed in this tooth form.

Labial surface analysis of the tooth form in Fig 2
The identifying characteristics of the labial surface of this tooth form are well-formed mesial and distal marginal ridges. However, these marginal ridges are not as prominent as those in Fig 4c. The proximal transitional surfaces are rather wide without significant difference between the width of the mesial and distal surfaces. A tooth with this form has prominent labial marginal ridges and prominent labial and proximal grooves. From the labial view, the mesioincisal and distoincisal line angles are both rounded, but the difference between them is clearly visible. In this form the labial accessory ridges, V-shaped grooves, transverse ridges, and grooves are well developed, and the surface characteristics are strong. Mamelon and perikymata are often present in this tooth form without any evidence of wear facets.

Labial surface analysis of the tooth form in Fig 3
The identifying characteristics of the labial surface of this tooth form are the nondescript marginal ridges that give the tooth an "expressionless" appearance. However, the central ridge is well developed and appears prominent from an incisal view. In this form of tooth, the labial grooves on both the mesial and distal aspects of the central ridge are rather visible, and they often extend to the cervical area. Both incisal line angles are angled and have no significant difference in shape. The transverse ridges and grooves are not well developed, and the surface is comparatively flat.

Characteristics of the Lingual Surface

Fig 5a

- Labioincisal ridge
- Escape route of the lingual fossa
- Incisal groove
- Linguo-incisal ridge
- Escape route of the lingual fossa
- Lingual fossa
- Proximal transitional surface

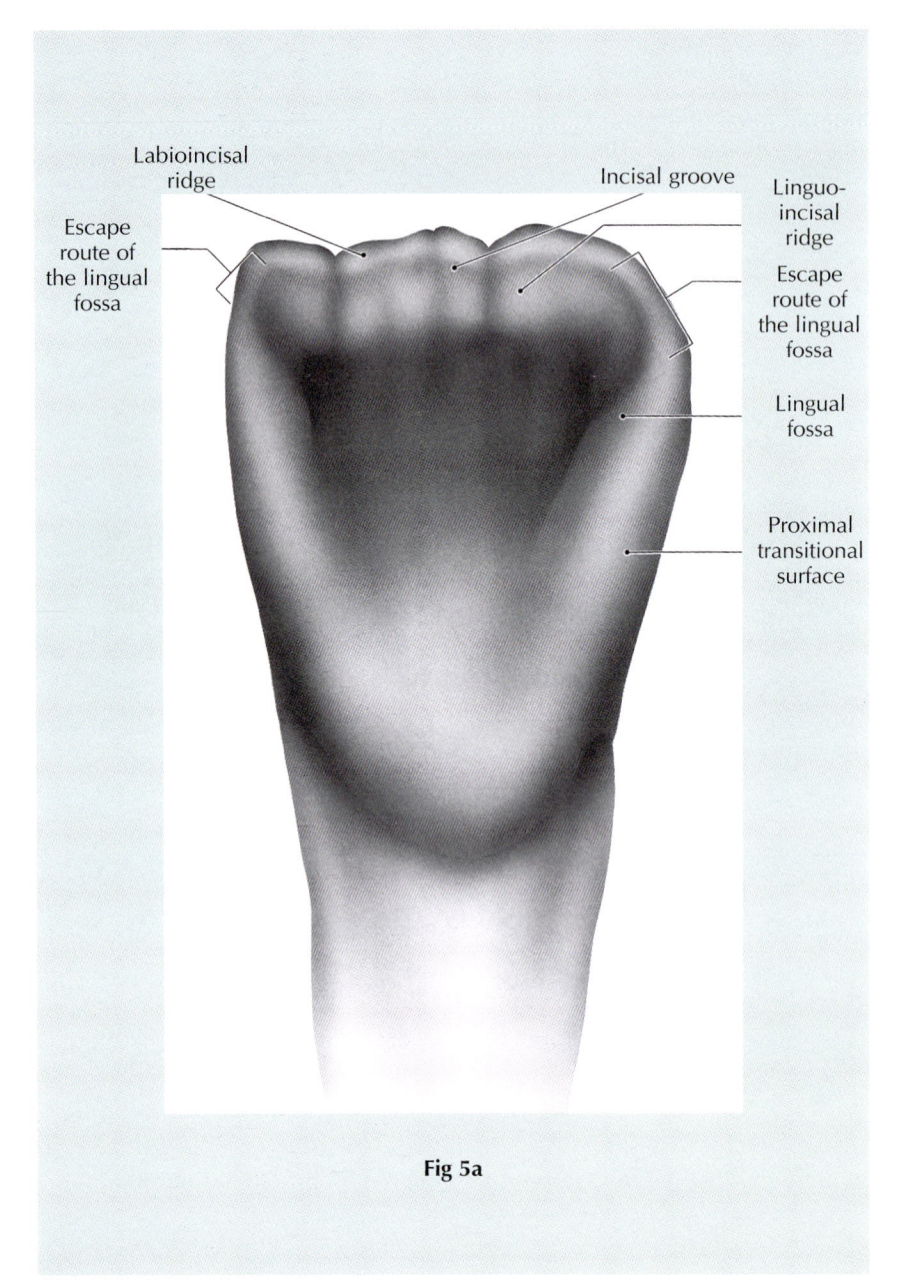

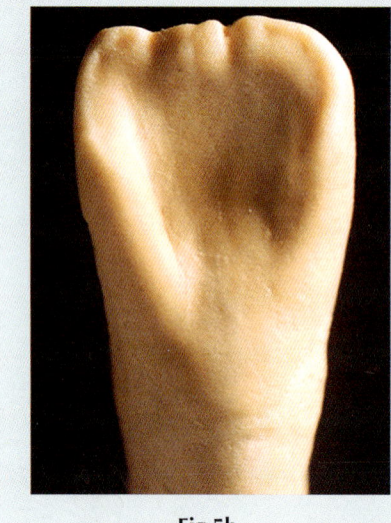

Fig 5b

The distinguishing features of the lingual surface of the tooth crown are well-developed mesial and distal marginal ridges and the surrounding triangular lingual fossa. The mesiolingual and distolingual marginal ridges extend to the cervical area and form a cingulum.

The mesiolingual marginal ridge extends high coronally toward the incisal edge, and the distolingual marginal ridge extends low cervically. The marginal ridges do not usually extend all the way to the incisal edge; therefore, the lingual fossa, which ends where the ridges end, also does not reach the incisal edge. The lingual fossa ends by exiting through the proximal areas at the "escape routes" of the lingual fossa.

Both the labioincisal ridge and the linguoincisal ridge are formed at the lingual aspect of the incisal area. They form an "incisal groove" that runs in a mesiodistal direction (see Fig 5b). The labioincisal ridge actually forms the shape of the incisal aspect of the tooth crown. The two incisal ridges and the incisal groove form the incisal slope that extends toward the lingual surface. The area that includes the incisal slope is where the "halo effect" can be detected. The halo effect is a characteristic of natural tooth color. The incisal ridges connect to the marginal ridges surrounding the escape routes of the lingual fossa.

A central ridge and accessory ridges are also present on the lingual surface. The degree of development of the central ridge affects the shape of the cingulum.

Fig 5c

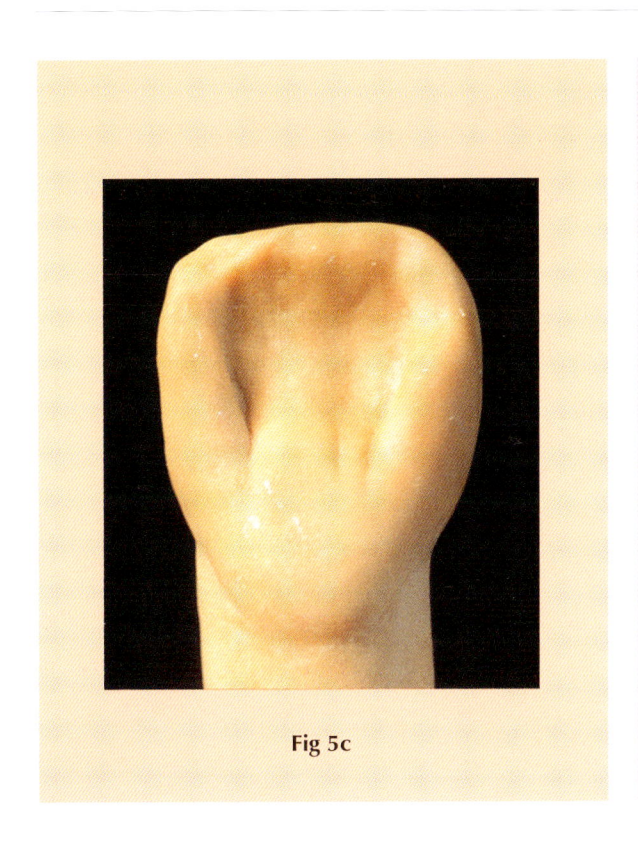

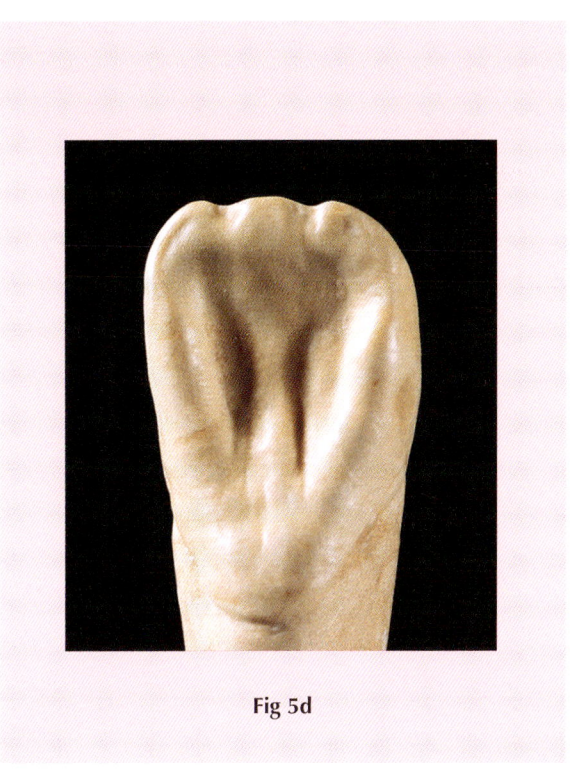

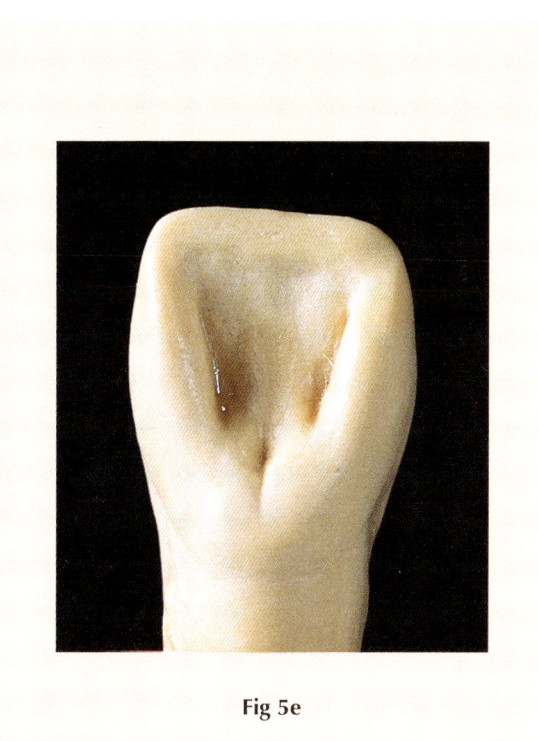

Fig 5d

Fig 5e

Lingual surface analysis of the tooth form in Fig 1
The identifying characteristics of the lingual surface of this tooth form are well-developed marginal ridges. The mesial marginal ridge extends to the incisal edge, but the distal marginal ridge does not and is rather short in comparison to the mesial. This is why the escape route of the lingual fossa is not present on the mesial aspect, but is wide on the distal. The lingual fossa is deep in proportion to the development of the marginal ridges, and the central and accessory ridges are not so prominent. The incisal ridge and groove are barely visible.

Lingual surface analysis of the tooth form in Fig 2
The identifying characteristics of the lingual surface of this type of tooth are that the marginal ridges are not as prominent as those in Fig 5c. Neither the mesial nor the distal marginal ridge extends to the incisal edge. The distal marginal ridge is shorter than the mesial marginal ridge. Since the marginal ridges do not extend to the incisal edge, the escape routes of the lingual fossa are visible on both marginal ridges. The distal escape route is a little wider than that on the mesial. The lingual central ridge is well developed and extends from the cingulum to the middle of the lingual surface. Since no wear facets are present, the incisal ridge and groove are prominent. The incisal groove, which extends to the developmental groove, is present on the incisal slope.

Lingual surface analysis of the tooth form in Fig 3
The identifying characteristics of the lingual surface of this tooth form are well-developed marginal ridges that narrow inward. The mesial and distal marginal ridges both extend to the incisal edge; thus, the escape route of the lingual fossa is not present on either side. The lingual fossa is deep in proportion to the development of the marginal ridges. The central and accessory ridges are not as prominent, but two spinous processes extend from the cingulum to the lingual fossa. Since the incisal edge of this tooth is worn, only a trace of the incisal groove is visible.

Characteristics of the Proximal Surfaces

Escape route of the lingual fossa

Proximal groove

Proximal transitional surfaces

Fig 6a

Fig 6b

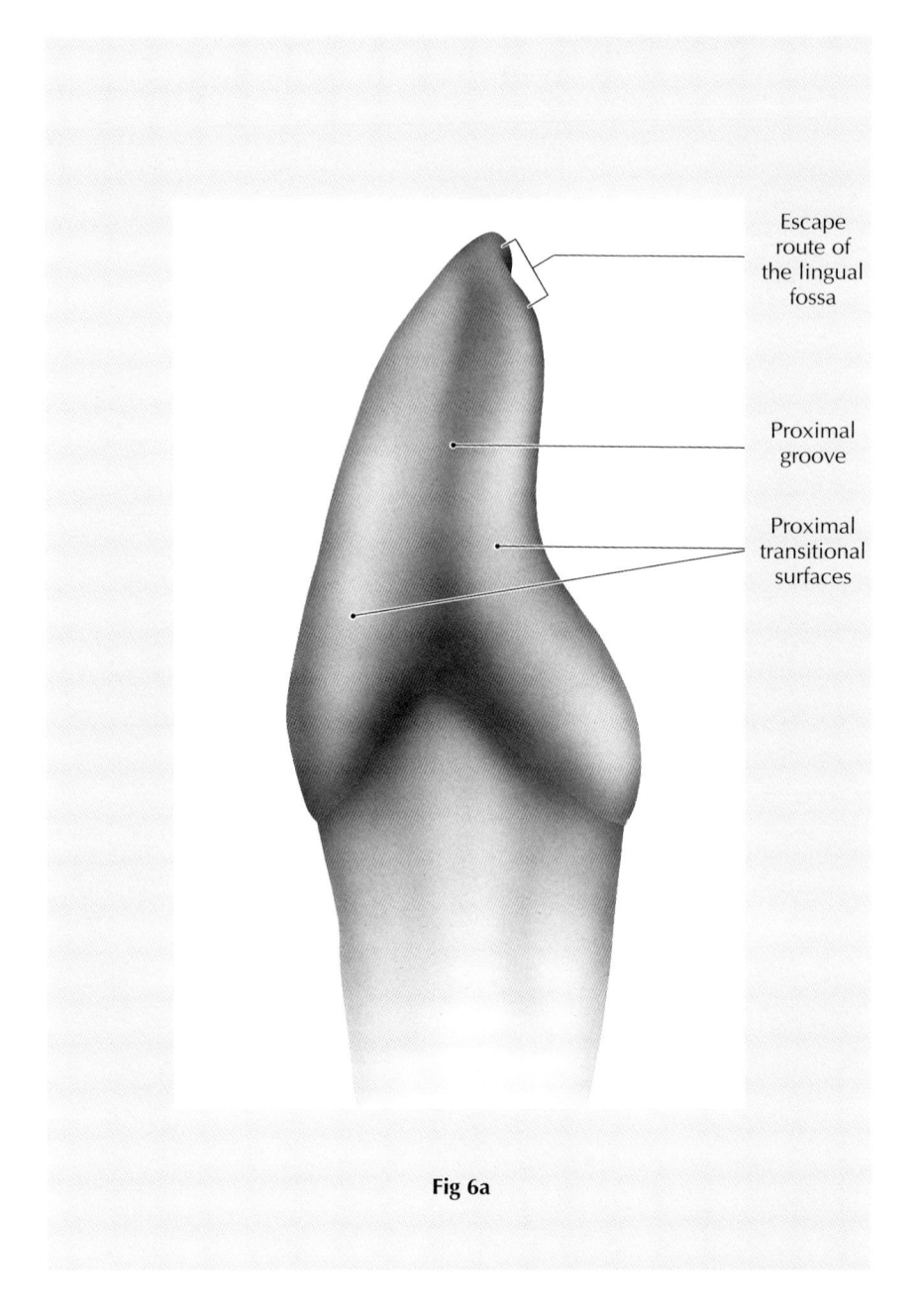

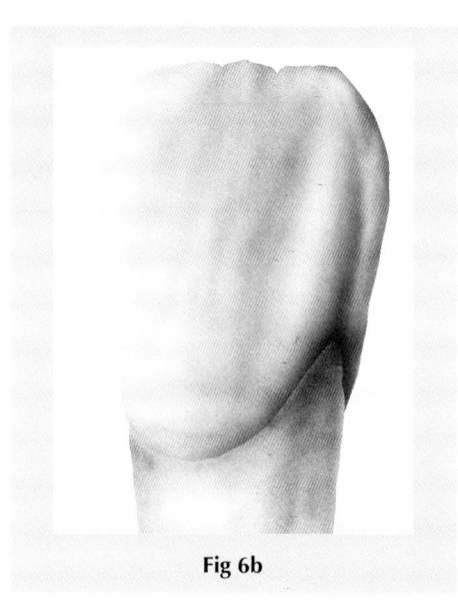

A tooth viewed from only the labial aspect may provide the false impression that marginal ridges exist only on the labial surface. However, marginal ridges should be considered and viewed as three-dimensional components that extend from the labial groove to the marginal inner slope, peak of the ridge, proximal transitional surface, and over to the middle of the proximal surface (Fig 6b). Thus, both the mesial and distal proximal surfaces consist of elevated parts, which are extensions of the labial and lingual marginal ridges toward the proximal area. A depression is formed where the labial and lingual marginal ridges meet. In this book, this depression is called the *proximal groove*. During the fabrication of a restoration, proper reproduction of the proximal groove is very important in creating the opening of the area of the line angles and the incisal interproximal space, which affect the tooth form.

The labiolingual location of the proximal groove at the incisal area is closely related to the escape route of the lingual fossa. Since the lingual marginal ridge ends at the point where the lingual fossa escapes to the proximal surface, this is where the labial and lingual marginal ridges meet; it is also the starting point of the proximal groove. A particular shape of depression is formed in this area. Since the mesiolingual marginal ridge extends high toward the incisal edge and the distolingual marginal ridge extends lower, the proximal groove is located toward the labial aspect on the mesial and toward the lingual aspect on the distal. In the proximal area, the cervical line extends high incisally (especially on the mesial side), and the proximal grooves run toward the peak of this cervical line.

Fig 6c

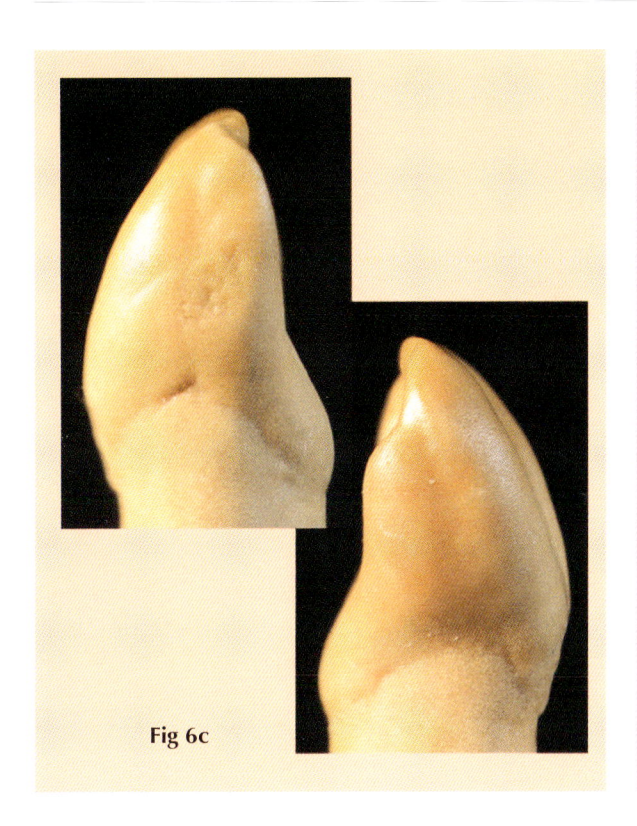

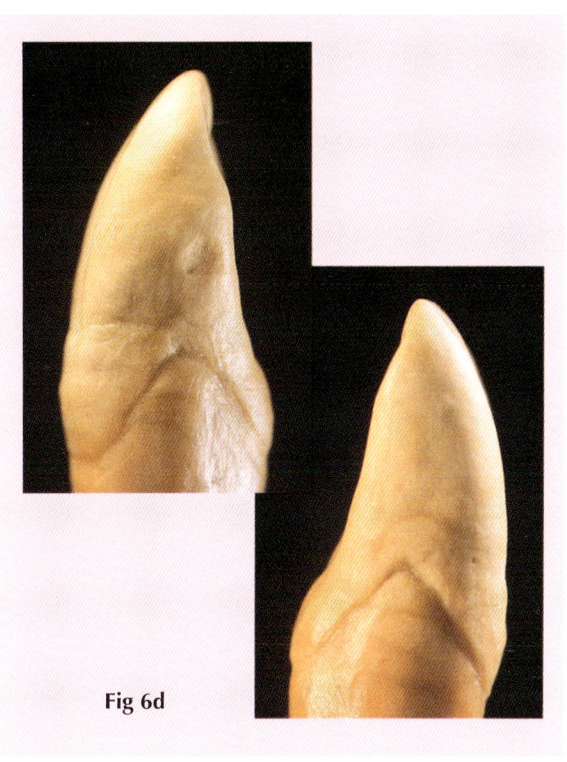

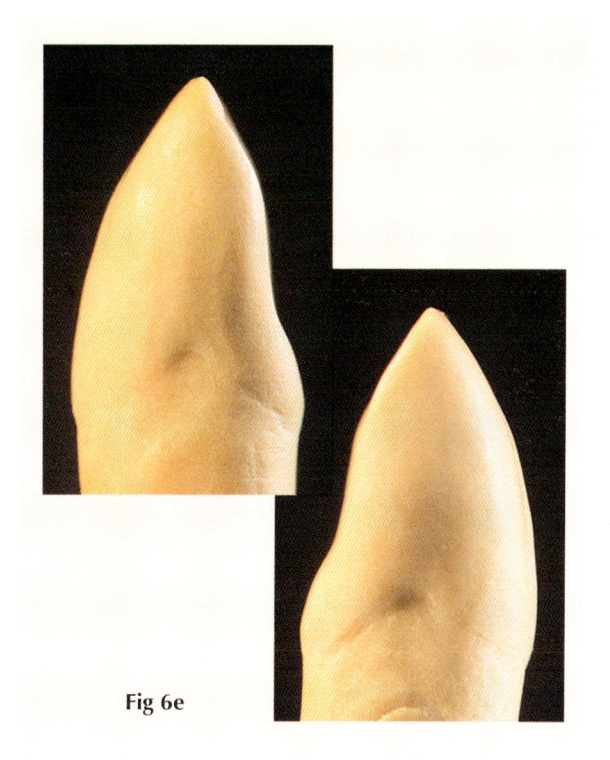

Fig 6d

Fig 6e

Proximal surface analysis of the tooth form in Fig 1
The mesial proximal surface of this tooth form is wide, and the proximal groove is deep because of the well-developed labial and lingual marginal ridges. Since the mesiolingual marginal ridge extends to the incisal edge, the proximal groove starts toward the labial side. The proximal groove runs toward the peak of the cervical line and is deeper in this area.

The distal proximal surface is similar to that on the mesial. However, because of the presence of the lingual fossa escape route, a strong depression is present. The proximal groove starts from this depression and runs in the middle or toward the lingual side of the proximal surface. In this type of tooth form, the cervical line extends high on the mesial side, but not as high on the distal.

Proximal surface analysis of the tooth form in Fig 2
The proximal surfaces of this tooth form are narrow, and the proximal grooves are shallow because of the poorly developed labial and lingual marginal ridges. The lingual marginal ridges do not reach the incisal edge on either the mesial or distal side; thus, the escape route of the lingual fossa is present on both the mesial and distal sides. The incisal edge tends to tip in toward the lingual side, and the cervical line extends high on both the mesial and distal sides.

Proximal surface analysis of the tooth form in Fig 3
The proximal surfaces of this tooth form are wide due to the well-developed lingual marginal ridges. However, because of the poorly developed labial marginal ridge, the proximal groove is not prominent, and the proximal surface is somewhat "expressionless." The lingual marginal ridges extend to the incisal edge on both sides; thus, the escape routes of the lingual fossa are not visible. Hence, a barely noticeable proximal groove is present in the middle of the proximal surface labiolingually. The cervical line does not extend high on either the mesial or distal side.

Transition Between Surfaces

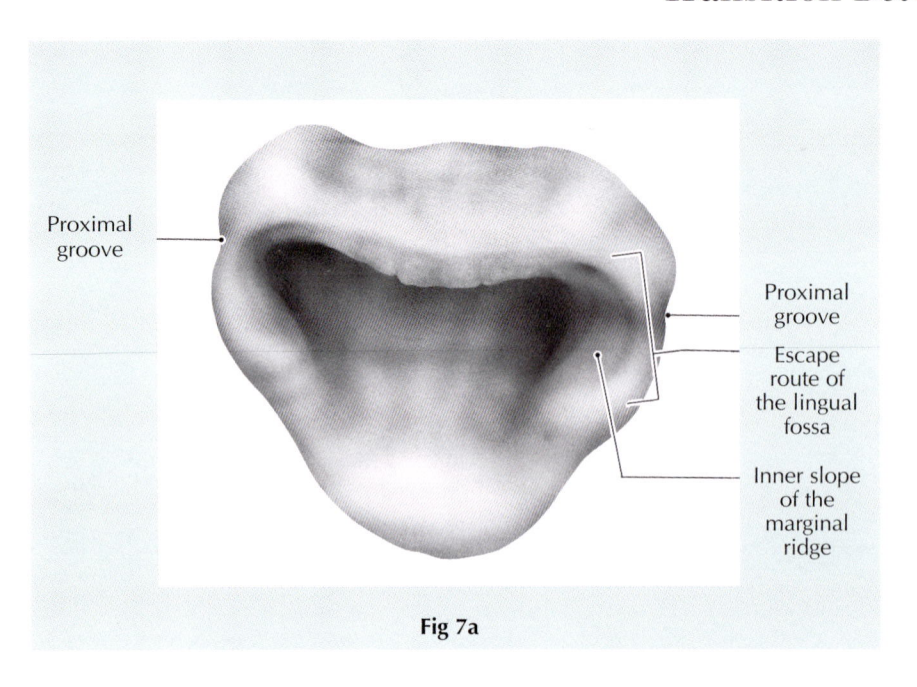

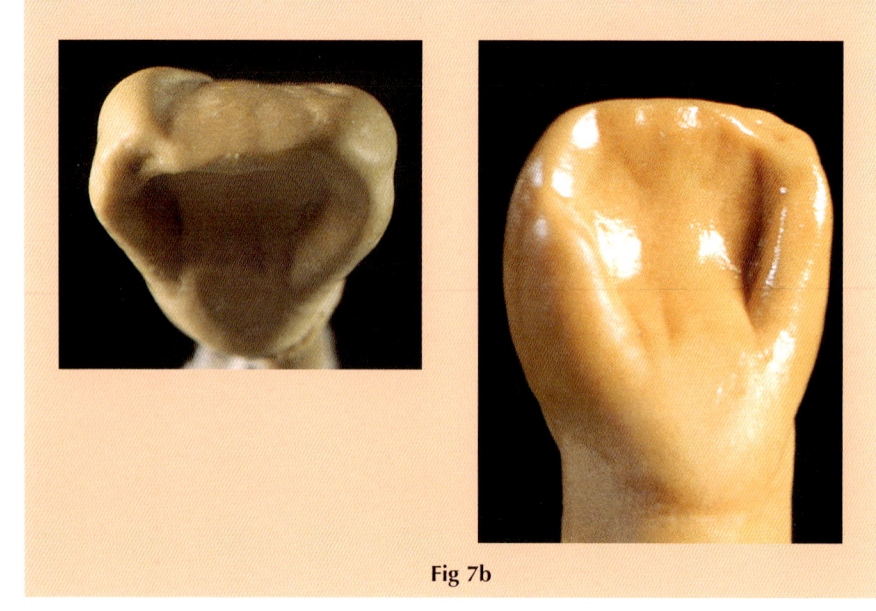

Fig 7a

Proximal groove
Proximal groove
Escape route of the lingual fossa
Inner slope of the marginal ridge

Fig 7b

The characteristics of the labial, lingual, and proximal surfaces have been analyzed separately; however, they are closely related to each other. To demonstrate this relationship, the proximal groove, the escape route of the lingual fossa, and the twist of the lingual marginal ridge are used as examples. On the labial and lingual surfaces, the incisal height of the marginal ridges is similar, as are the position and direction of the central or accessory ridge. This similarity exists simply because both originate from the same developmental lobes and the developmental grooves are connected labiolingually at the incisal edge (Figs 7a to 7d).

As mentioned in the discussion on the characteristics of the proximal surfaces, a marginal ridge is a three-dimensional composition that consists of the inner slope of the ridge, peak of the ridge, proximal transitional surface, and half of the proximal surface on the labial and lingual sides. Thus, the proximal grooves and the lingual grooves are the result of the development of the labial and lingual marginal ridges (see Figs 6c and 6d), and the degree of development of those ridges determines the position and depth of these grooves. The lingual marginal ridges usually do not extend to the incisal edge, and therefore form the escape routes of the lingual fossa. The escape routes consist of twisted planes due to projection of the lingual marginal ridges. This area is the border of the labial and the lingual marginal ridges; the proximal groove and the lingual groove are connected in this area. One might therefore think that the labial and lingual marginal ridges are separated, but the peak of the lingual marginal ridge is in fact connected to the labial marginal ridge (Figs 7a to 7d).

Fig 7c

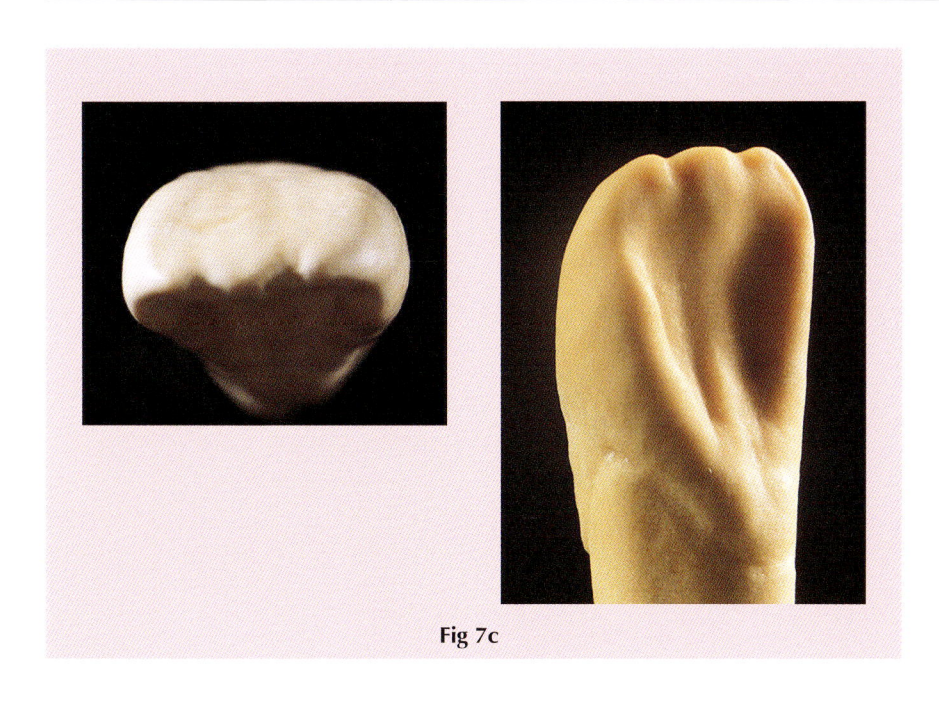

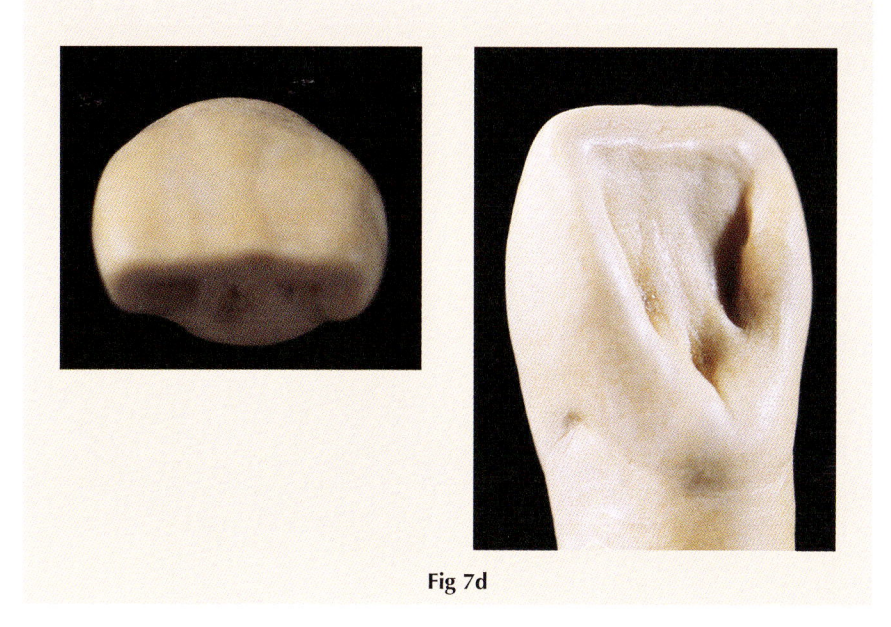

Fig 7d

A comparison of the mesiolingual and distolingual marginal ridges shows that the mesial marginal ridge is narrower and extends higher toward the incisal edge. Since the mesial ridge is not as twisted as the distal ridge and the area of the inner slope is smaller, the projection of the peak of the mesial ridge is small and creates a straight image. On the other hand, the distal ridge is shorter and thicker. Since it is strongly twisted and the area of the inner slope is wider, the peak of the ridge is projected vigorously and creates a round image (Figs 7a to 7d).

The escape route of the lingual fossa and the transition of the peak from the lingual marginal ridge to the labial marginal ridge are closely related to the labial image of the mesial and distal line angles. Because of the escape route of the lingual fossa, the labial marginal ridge, especially the labiodistal marginal ridge, collapses toward the lingual side, and this collapse makes the distoincisal line angle round. On the other hand, the mesioincisal line angle is angled. Figures 4c to 4e demonstrate this relationship well. Moreover, since the lingual marginal ridge projects with some twisting, the lingual side is wider than the labial side, and the lingual marginal ridge is visible behind the labial marginal ridge in the labial view. Therefore, the projection of the lingual marginal ridge and the way the peak is connected to the labial marginal ridge affect the labial image of the incisal line angles. These two factors also affect the width and the angle of the proximal transitional surface of the labial marginal ridges and determine the proportion between the overall width of the tooth crown and the width of the labial surface. They are important factors in the characteristics of labial tooth form.

Thus, as one can clearly see, tooth-surface compositions affect each other, and a thorough understanding of the relationship between tooth surfaces is essential to fabricate a natural-looking ceramic restoration.

Reproduction of the Form with Well-Developed Marginal Ridges

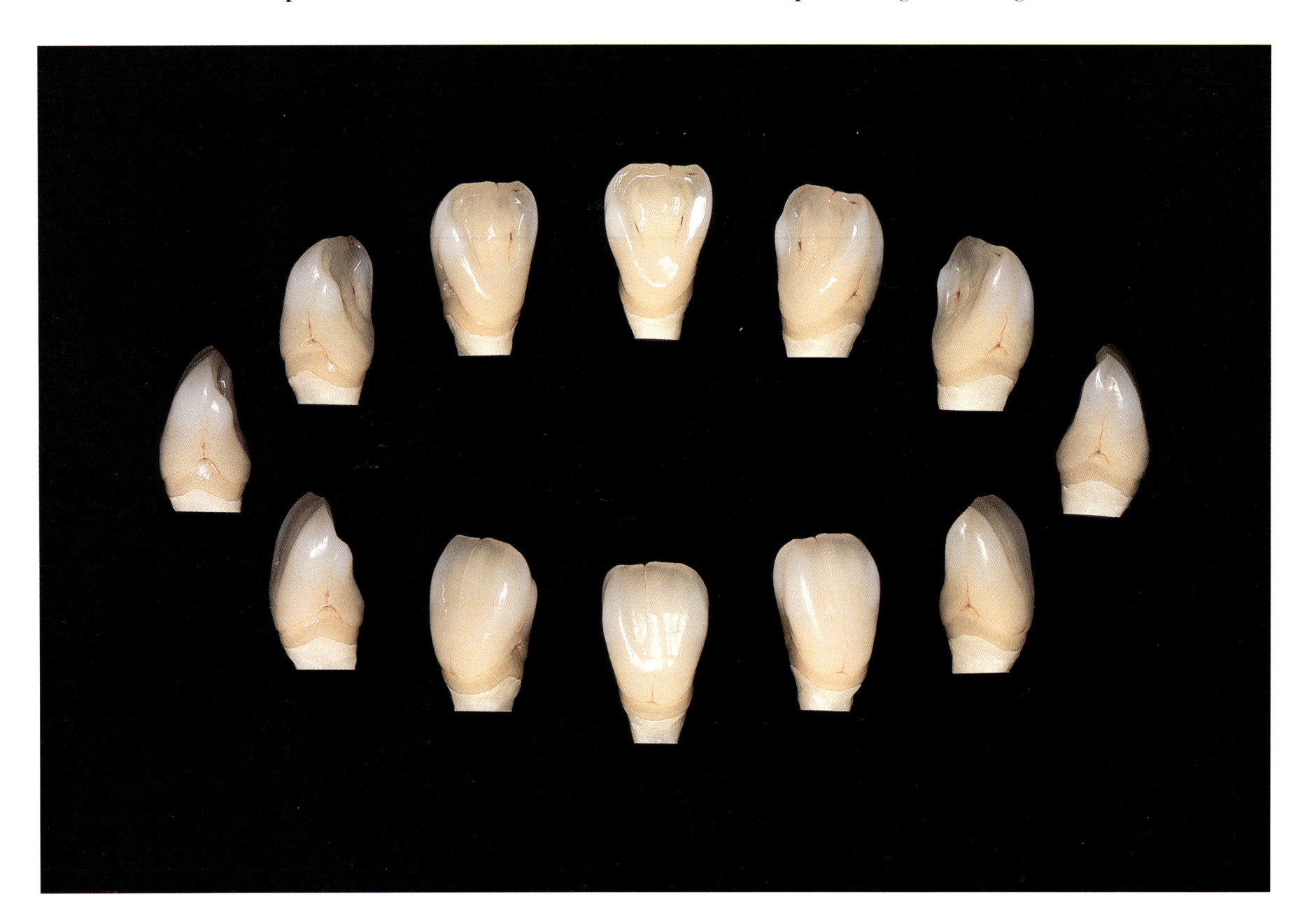

Transition to successive teeth

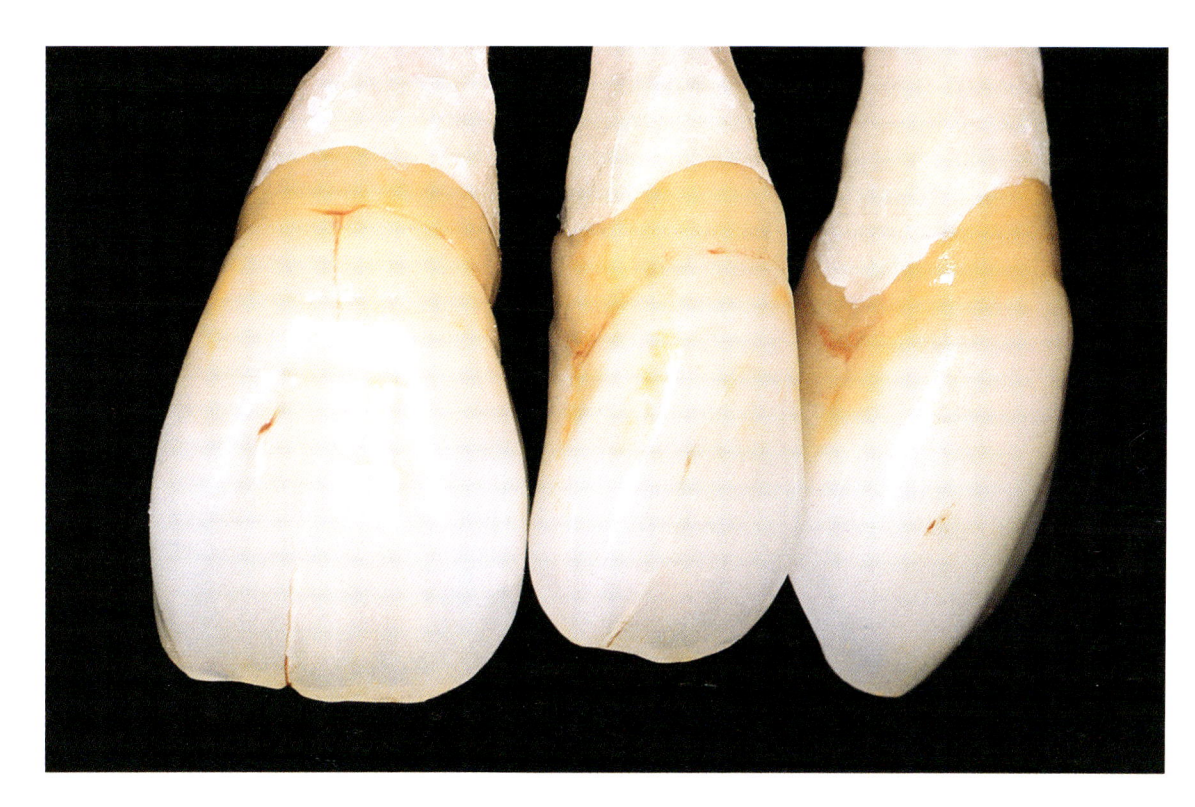

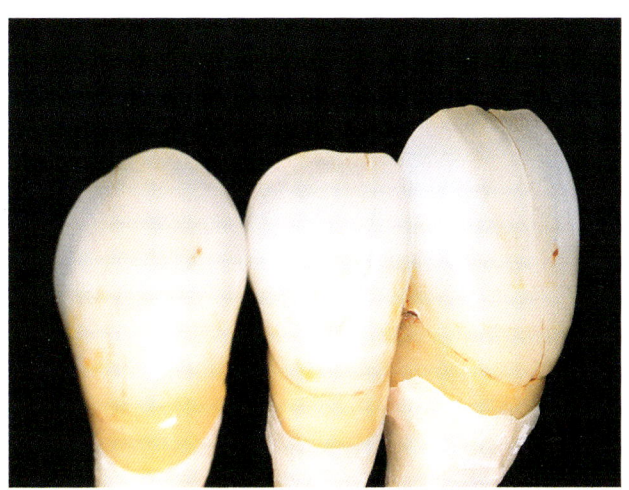

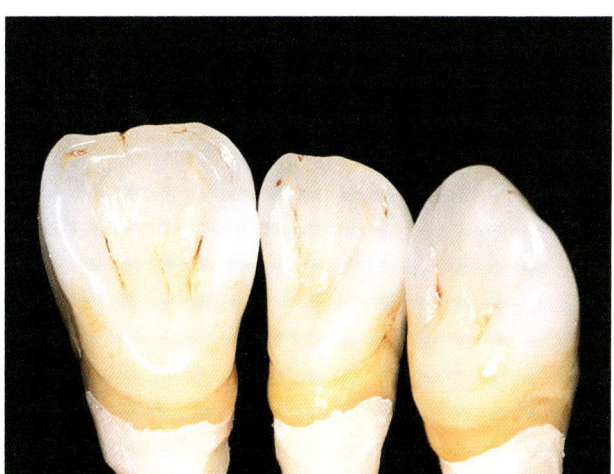

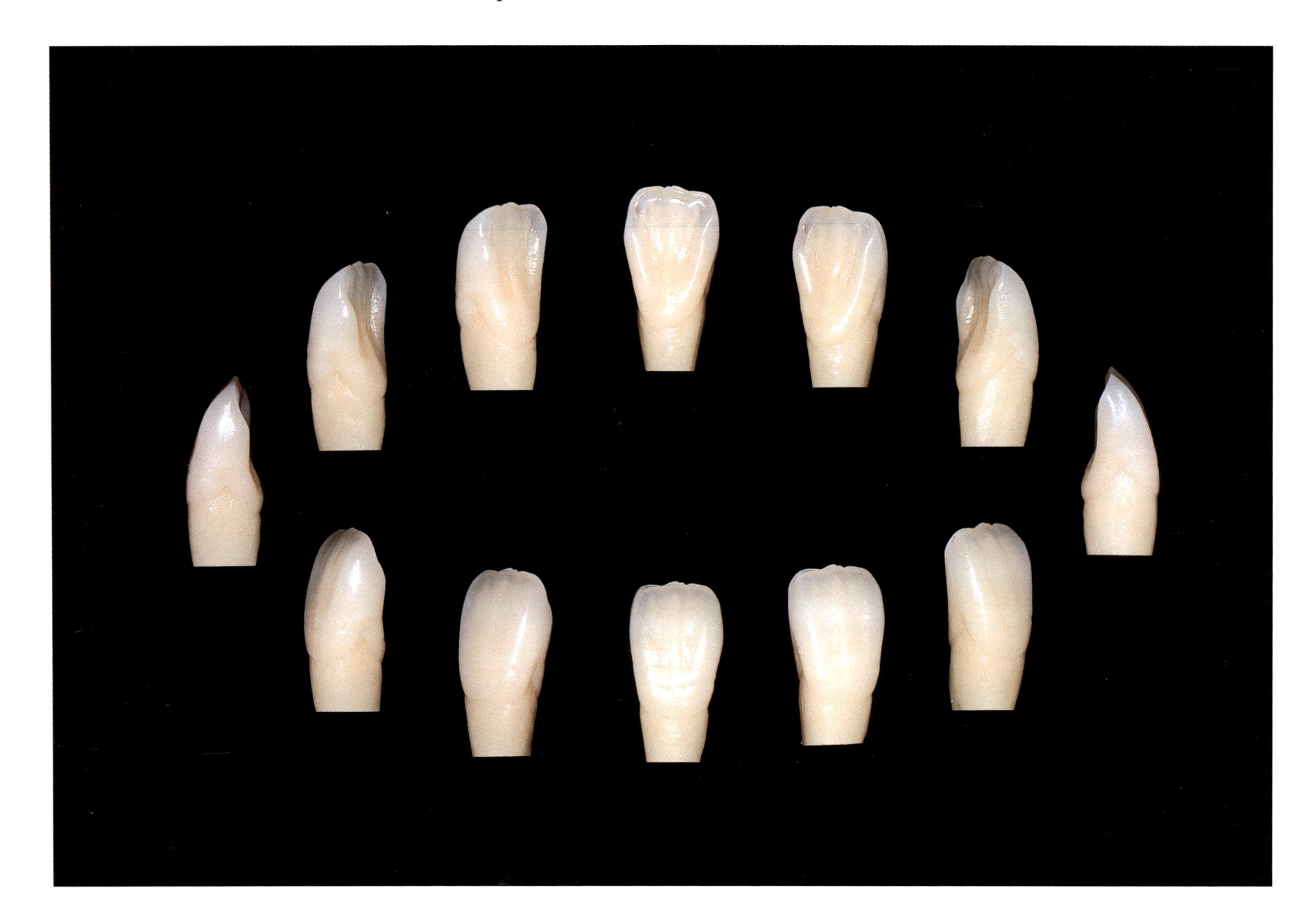

Reproduction of the Basic Form

Transition to successive teeth

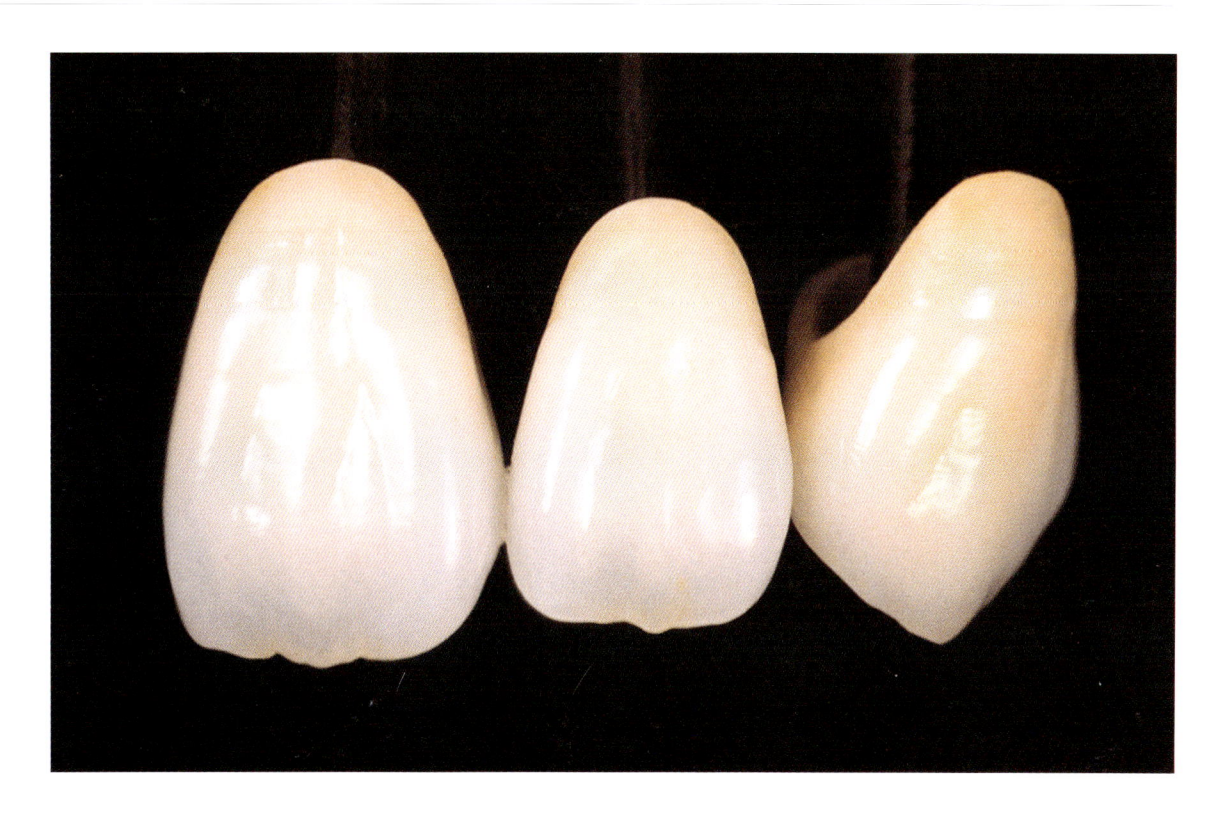

ch 2 | 41

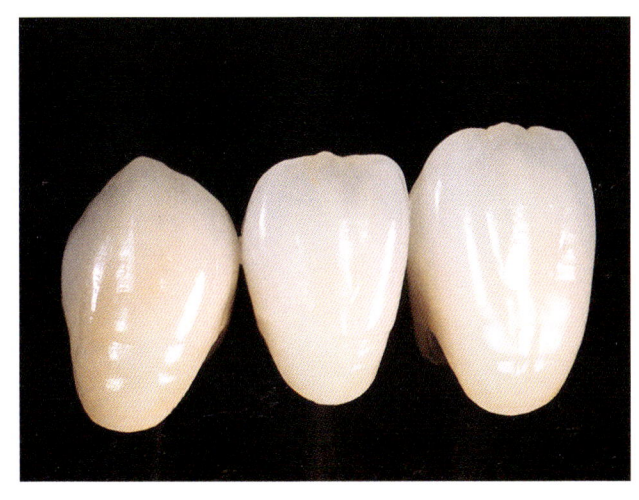

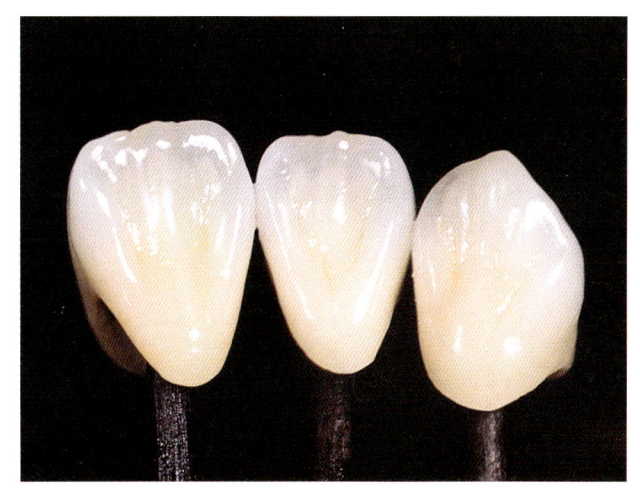

Reproduction of the Form Without Particular Characteristics

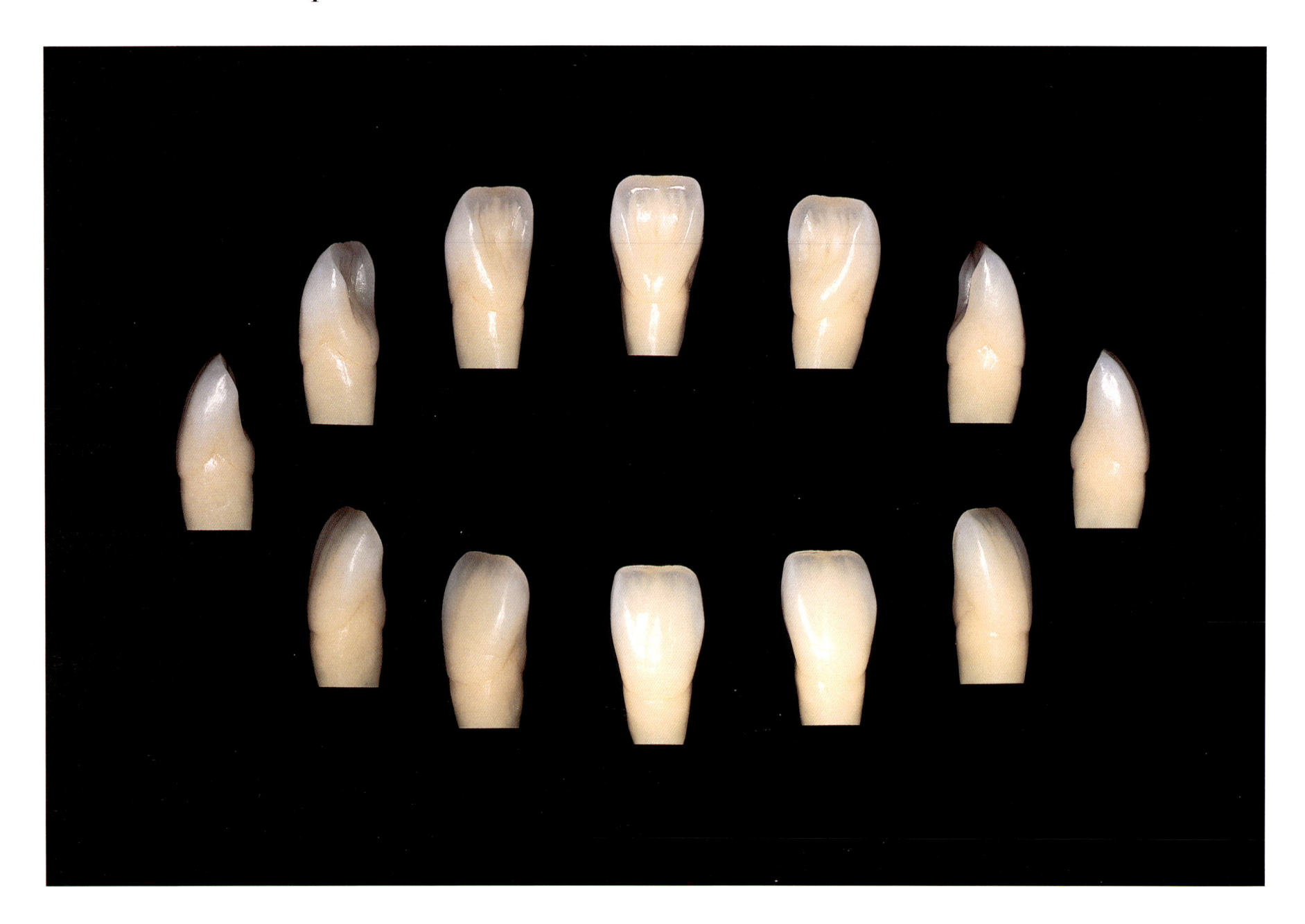

Transition to successive teeth

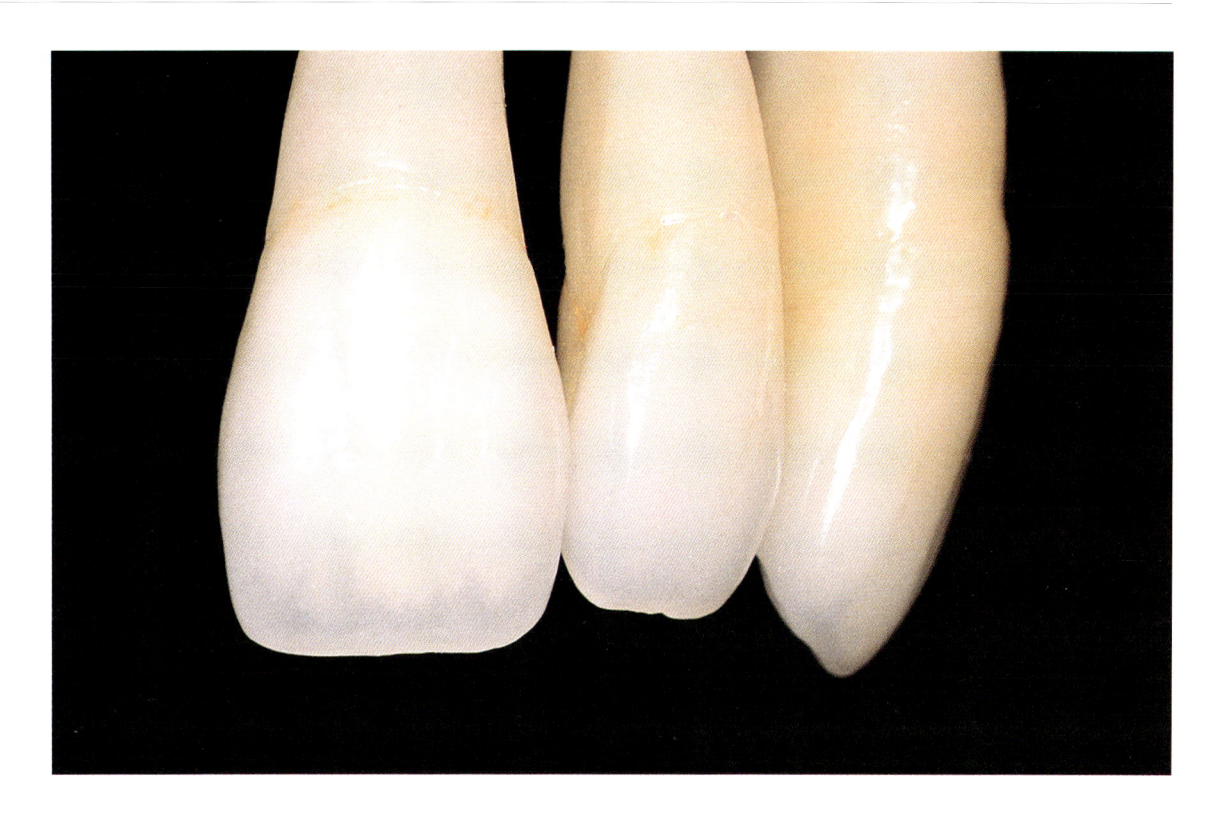

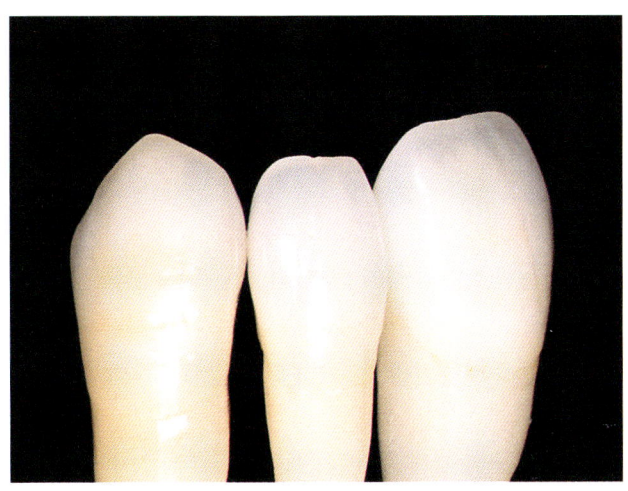

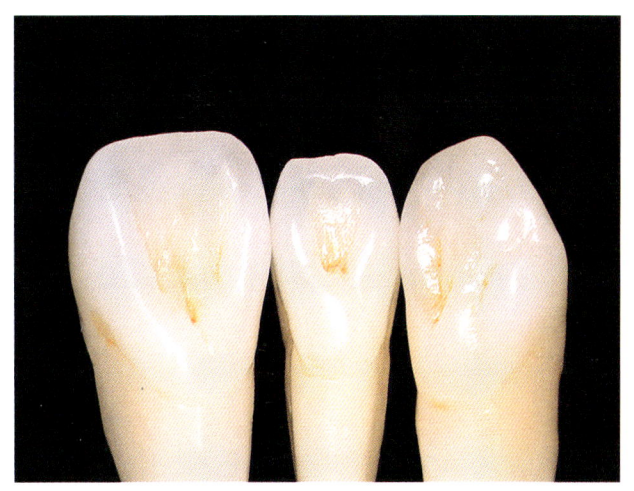

CHAPTER 3

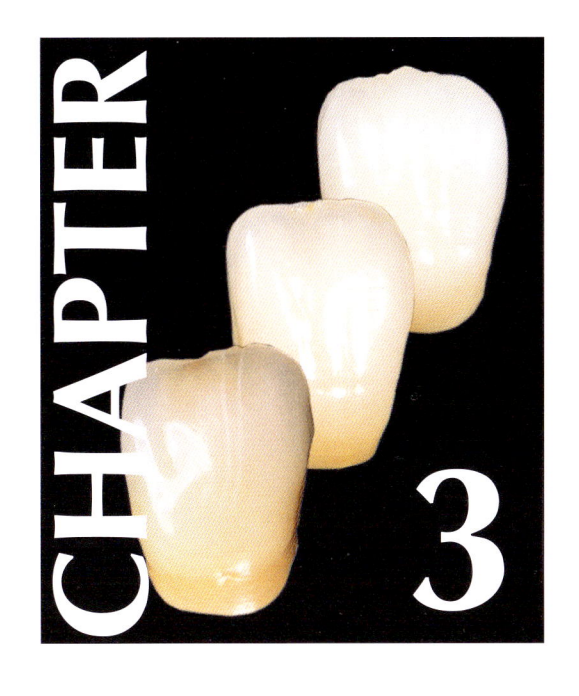

The Effect of Aging on Tooth Morphology

Changes in Tooth Appearance

It is important to fabricate ceramic restorations with shape and color that appropriately reflect the patient's age.

In chapter 1 the three basic shapes of tooth crown morphology were discussed independently of extrinsic factors. However, in the oral environment, extrinsic factors, such as changes in the supporting periodontal apparatus and wear facets, affect tooth appearance; thus, the processes that occur during aging strongly affect the appearance of the tooth.

The anatomic cervical line is located subgingivally during adolescence; therefore, the clinical cervical line is coronal to the anatomic cervical line. As a result, in adolescents the morphology of the visible tooth crown is commonly ovoid or square. With age, periodontal tissue undergoes degenerative change. First the anatomic cervical line, then the root, are exposed, and the visible cervical aspect gradually narrows in comparison with that of the young dentition. In addition, the incisal edge area will be worn down over the years, and the round incisal line angles will become acute. Thus, the clinical crowns seen during adolescence, which are square or ovoid in shape, become tapered with age due to the combination of cervical crown exposure and incisal edge wear.

In adolescence, the surface characteristics (eg, labial accessory ridges, V-shaped grooves, and perikymata) are obvious, and the surface appears rough. As teeth age, their surface texture will change noticeably due to continuous abrasion and attrition. As a result, the rough surface texture that characterizes the young tooth will become shiny and smooth.

Aging also affects tooth color, mainly due to the increased reflection of the color of the dentin through the labial surfaces. Over the years accumulated calcification increases the translucency of the enamel, enabling the color of dentin to gradually increase its reflection through the labial enamel. During adolescence, the dentinal color is blocked by enamel of low translucency. Changes in aging dentin itself also affect tooth color. High diffusion of light by primary dentin decreases with age, and progression of dentinal translucency changes the tooth color from an opaque light color to a translucent dark color. Because of these factors, the high-value whitish color of the adolescent tooth changes to a low-value orange, then to a low-value brownish color with age.

It is the authors' belief that in esthetic restorations, changes in tooth morphology and the color of enamel and dentin should be expressed realistically according to the patient's age. Attempting to create the illusion of aging in a restoration by mere surface staining, rather than by reproducing the internal changes in the aged dentition, may significantly decrease the esthetic outcome.

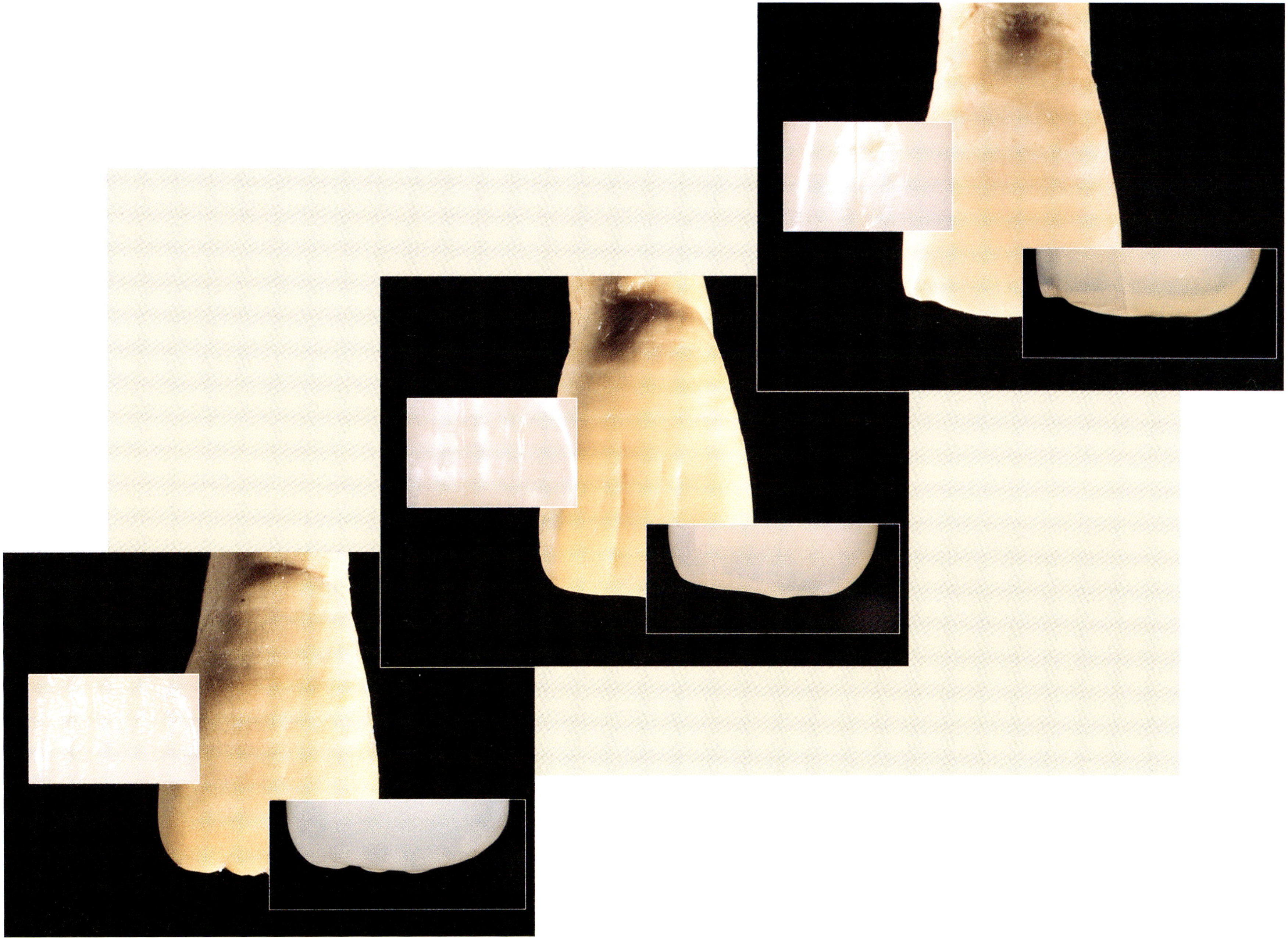

Extrinsic Factors that Affect the Appearance of Tooth Crowns

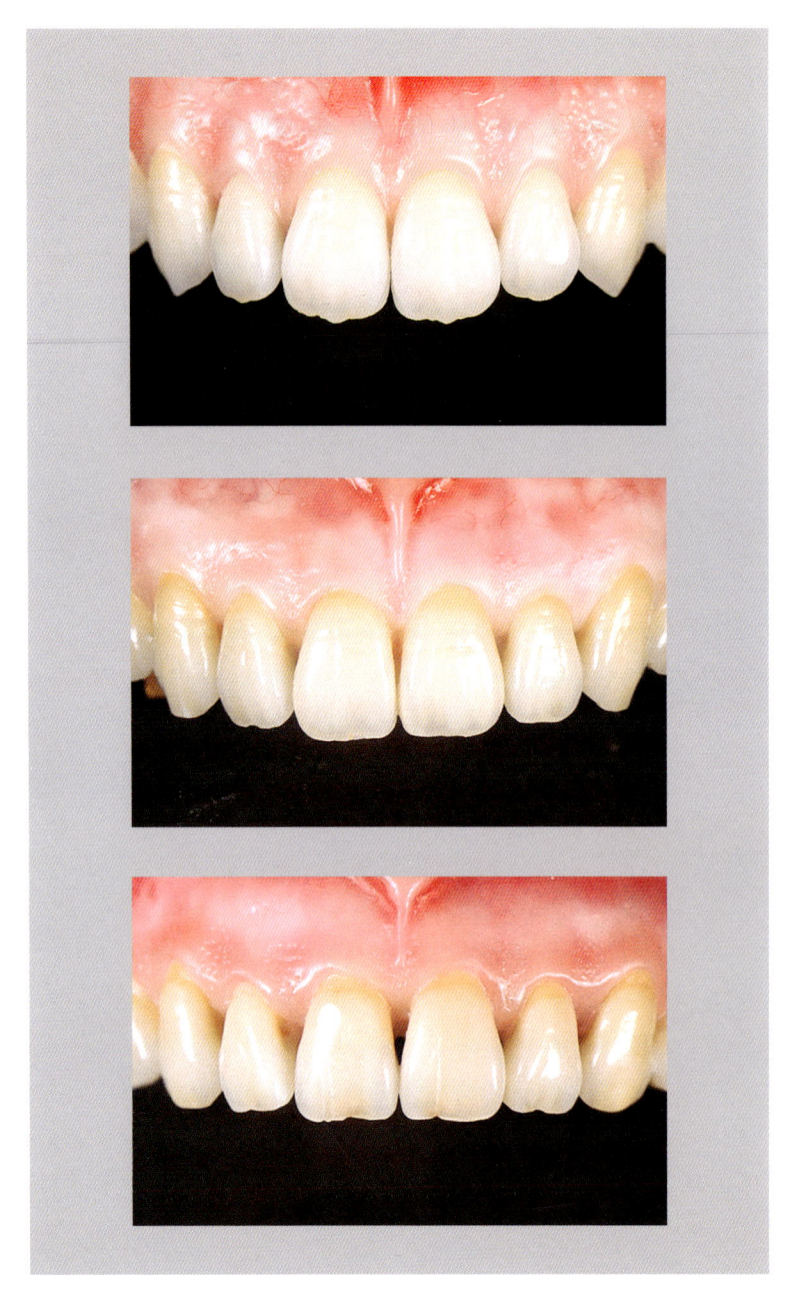

Changes in tooth morphology

Due to incomplete eruption, the clinical crown of the adolescent does not display the anatomic cervical line. This line is located subgingivally, and the clinical cervical line is located coronally to the anatomic cervical line. The gingival apparatus covers the narrow anatomic cervical line in the adolescent, and the clinical crown appears square or ovoid.

Teeth reveal their morphologic shape only after complete eruption. Aging will expose the anatomic cervical line, then the root surface. This exposure of the narrowed cervical area, in conjunction with the continuous reduction of the rounded incisal line angles due to abrasion and attrition, will result in teeth that appear tapered regardless of their original basic shape.

Changes in the incisal edge

Mamelons are usually clearly visible during adolescence, but they disappear at a relatively early age due to attrition. As the effects of attrition progress with age, incisal edges are gradually shortened and flattened. The incisal edges will present various kinds of wear patterns depending on the existing occlusal scheme.

Due to the horizontal and vertical overlap of the dentition, wear facets appear on the lingual surfaces of the maxillary anterior dentition and on the labial surfaces of the mandibular anterior dentition. Because the wear facets of the maxillary anterior teeth are not visible from the labial view, the only visible change is the gradual shortening of the incisal edges. In worn surfaces, dentin may become exposed over time, especially at the incisal edge. Because dentin is softer than enamel, it wears faster, and a depression can be created in the incisal edge. Exposed dentin will also be stained. This pattern of incisal wear facets and color variation should be properly reproduced in the esthetic restoration.

Changes in incisal edge alignment of the maxillary anterior dentition

In the intact maxillary anterior dentition of the adolescent, central incisor crowns are 1 to 2 mm longer than those of lateral incisors, and canines are as long as the central incisors or slightly longer. Attrition begins with function and is first evident in the canines, which are usually flattened by middle age.

Attrition manifestation then progresses to the central incisors, in which attrition begins at the middle part of the tooth and moves toward the mesial and distal line angles. Attrition is manifested last in the lateral incisors. In many instances, by middle age the central incisors, lateral incisors, and canines may be leveled.

In the elderly person, the central incisors and canines may be completely flattened. It is then when attrition starts to affect the incisal edges of the lateral incisors. The incisal line of the maxillary anterior dentition becomes rather straight. It is important to reproduce these changes of the incisal alignment in ceramic restorations.

Changes in surface texture

In the adolescent, the surface characteristics of teeth, such as labial accessory ridges, V-shaped grooves, and perikymata, are well developed, and the surface texture is rough. Over time, surfaces become flat and shiny due to abrasion by toothbrushing. It is important to reproduce this age-dependent change of surface texture in ceramic restorations.

Note: The realistic reproduction of an exposed root surface and attrition in the restoration is very effective in expressing age. However, the reproduction of the incisal characteristics should not hinder the establishment of proper occlusion.

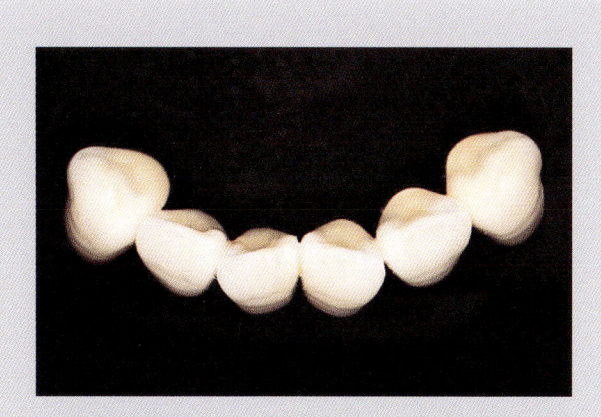

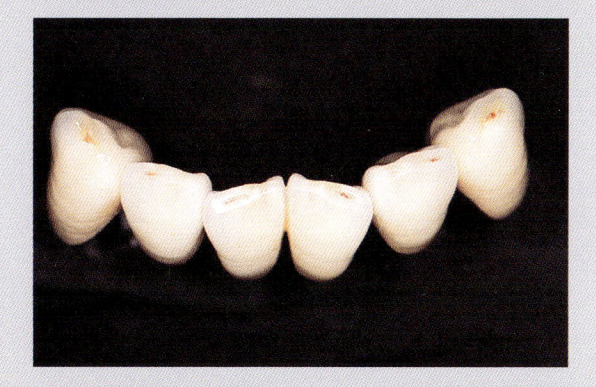

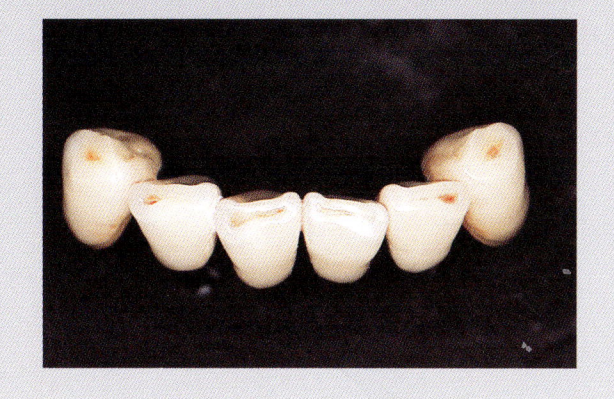

Expression of Changes in Tooth Morphology and Dentition with Age

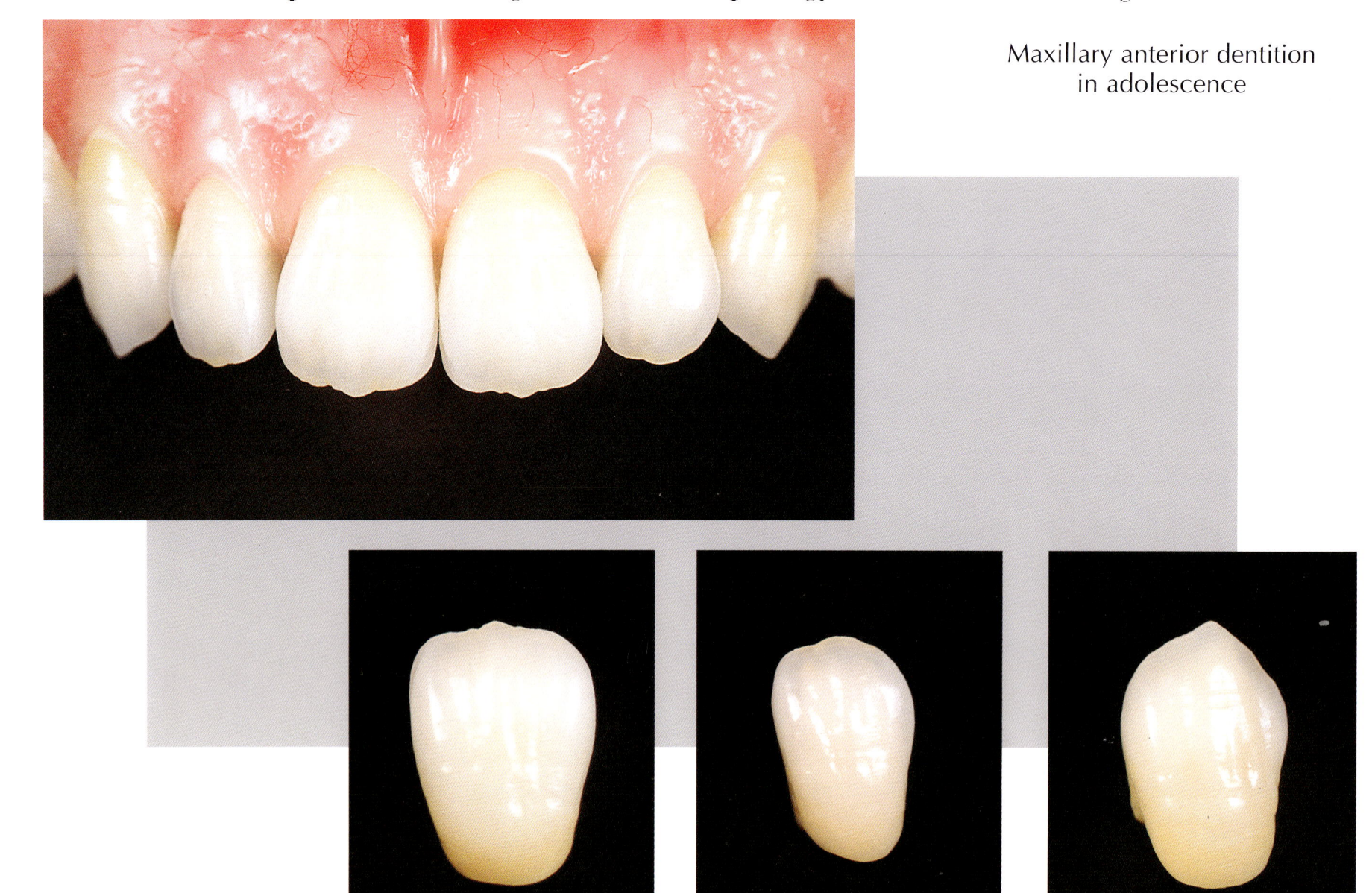

Maxillary anterior dentition in adolescence

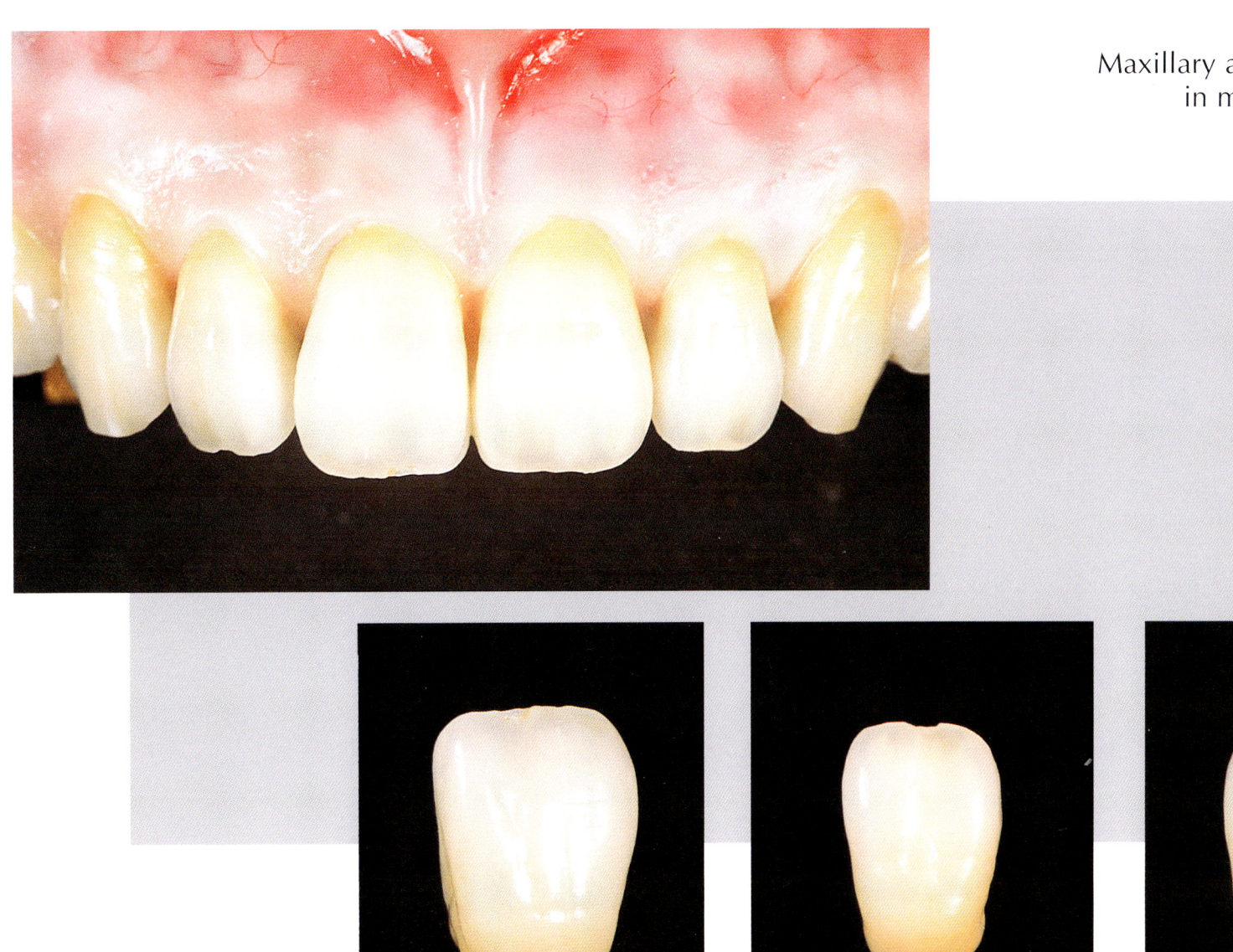

Maxillary anterior dentition
in middle age

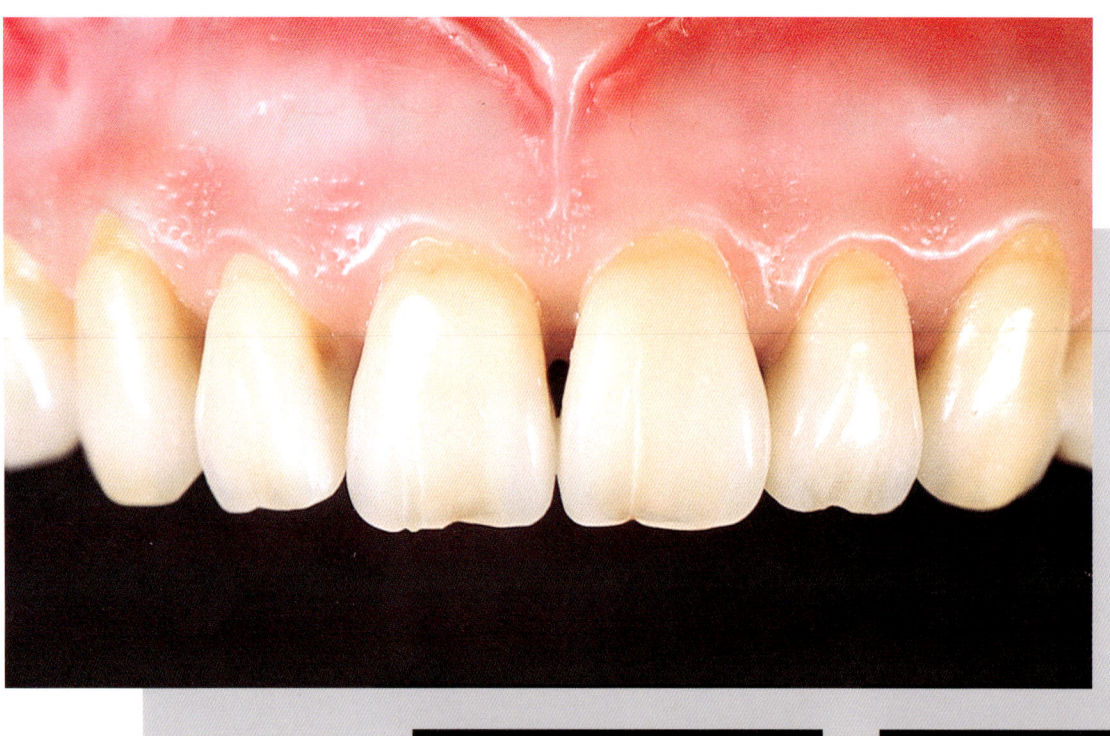

Maxillary anterior dentition
in old age

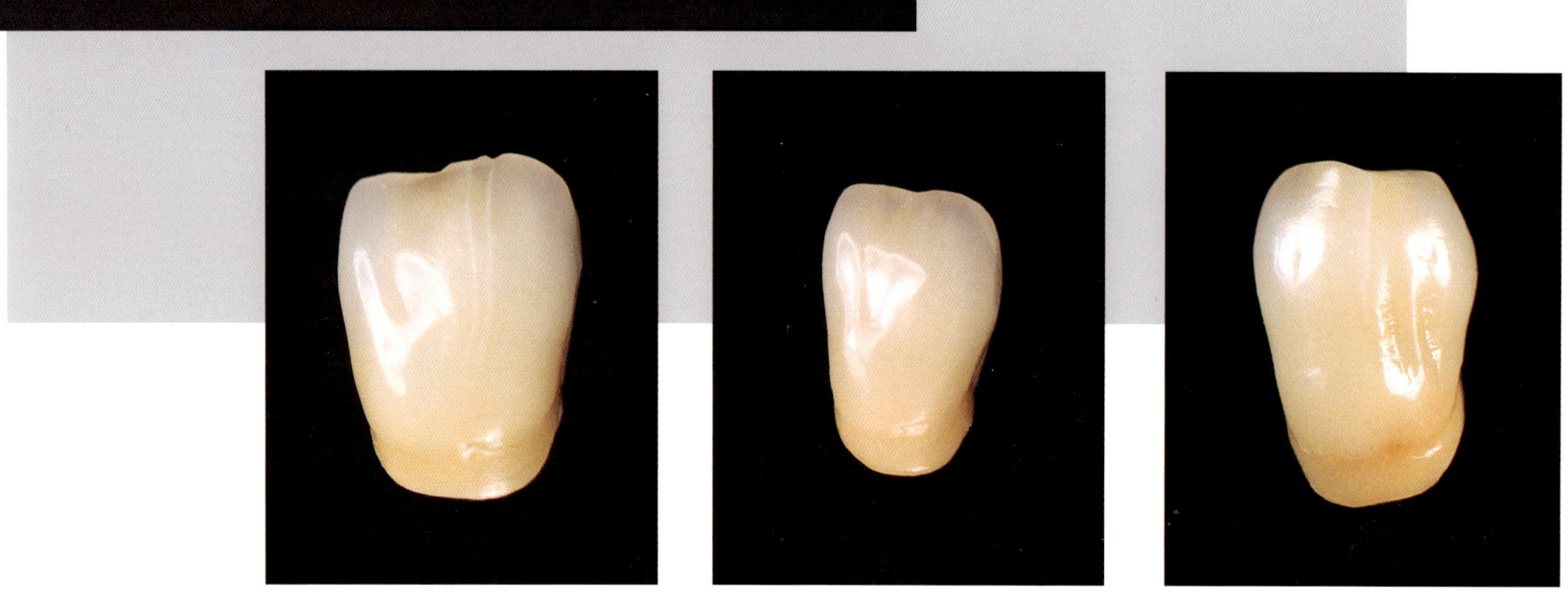

Mandibular anterior dentition

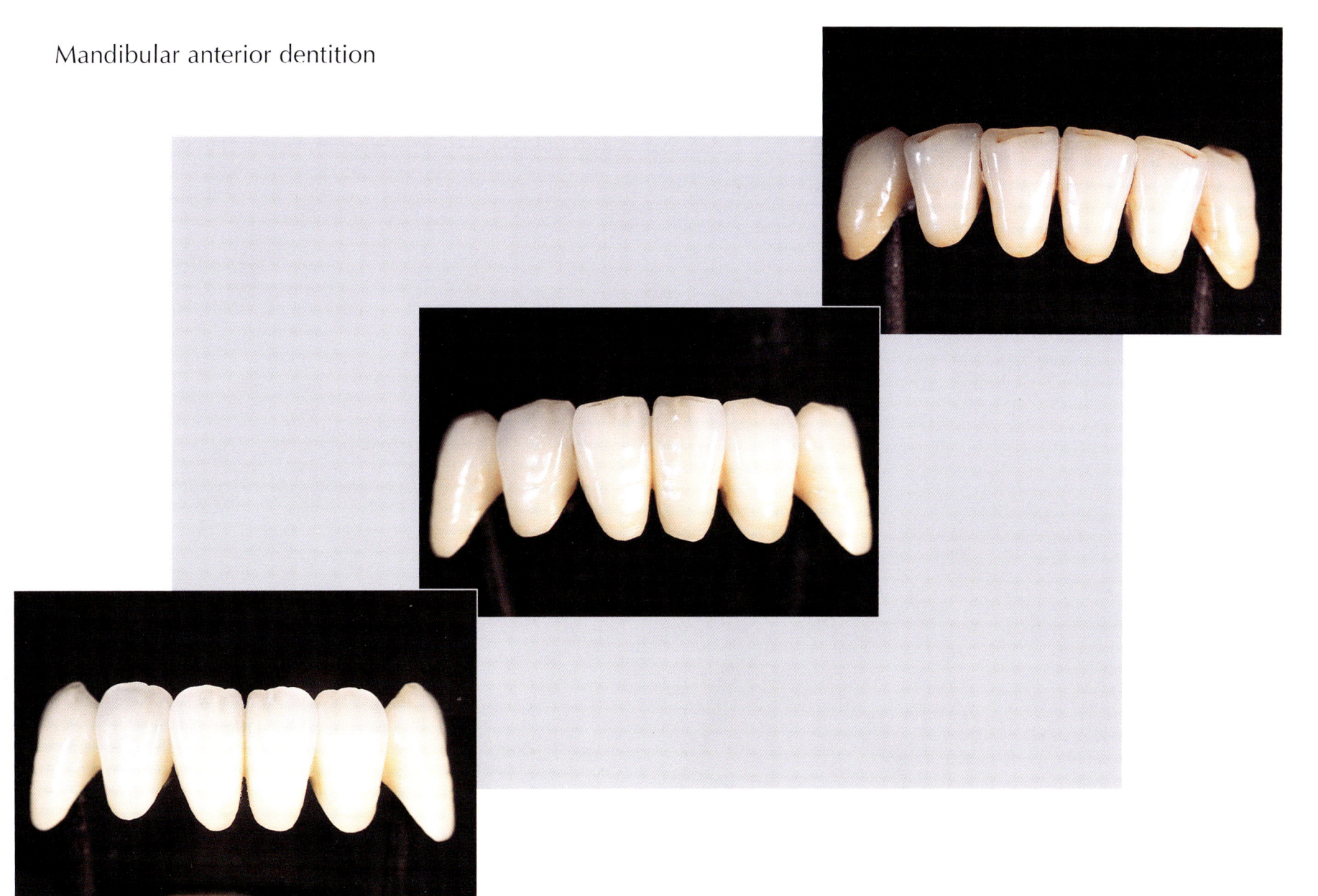

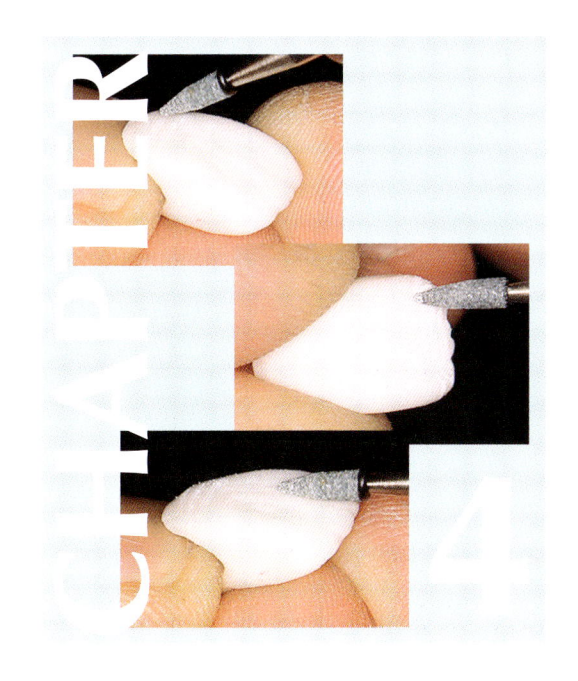

Contouring Ceramic Restorations I

Contouring a Single Restoration

In addition to understanding tooth morphology—the three basic shapes, variation of forms, and their interrelationship as discussed in chapters 1 and 2—one should be able to envision the complex as a whole; otherwise, it is difficult to understand where and how to contour a ceramic restoration and to reproduce the three-dimensional composition of natural teeth. After one understands natural tooth morphology as a complex, it is possible to fabricate esthetic ceramic restorations that harmonize with the supporting periodontal apparatus and the existing natural teeth.

Contouring of ceramic restorations is not achieved by the process of addition, or buildup, but by reduction. The ceramist reduces the fired, oversized porcelain to the proper, final shape.

Ceramic restorations consist of layers of porcelain with opaque, dentin, enamel, and translucent colors and are designed to create a composition that mimics the color and shape of the natural tooth. In porcelain-fused-to-metal restorations, cutting back the full-contour waxup of the tooth form shapes the metal framework. This framework is considered to be one layer within the composition of the restoration.

Maintaining the proper sequence of each contouring and finishing step is important to achieve the desired definitive shape of the restoration. Furthermore, proper instrument selection and modification, if necessary, are important to reproduce accurate shape and surface texture.

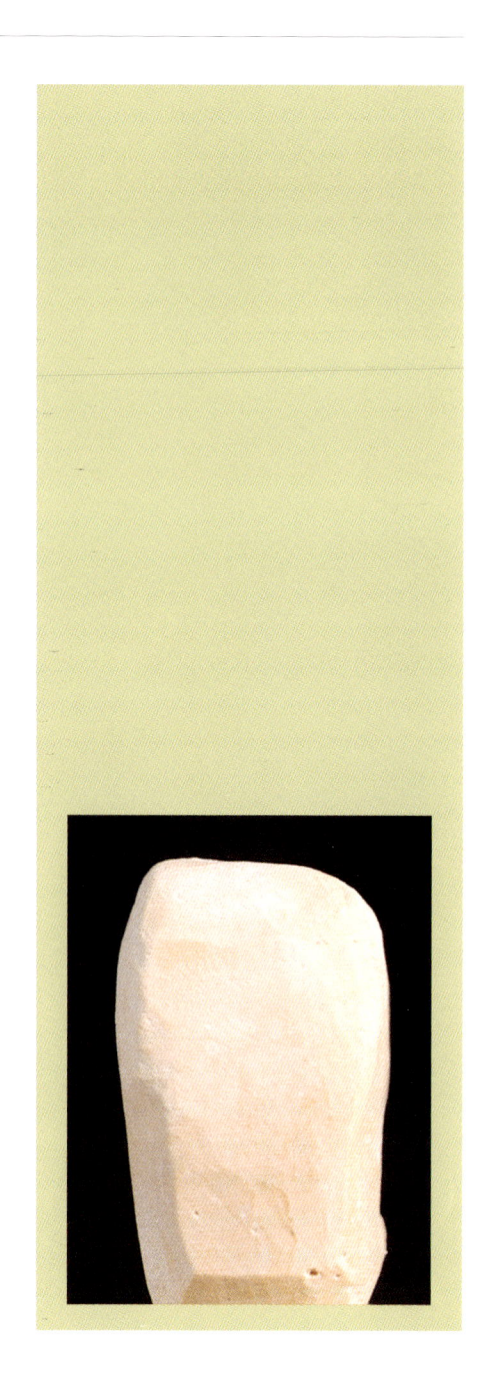

ch 4 | 57

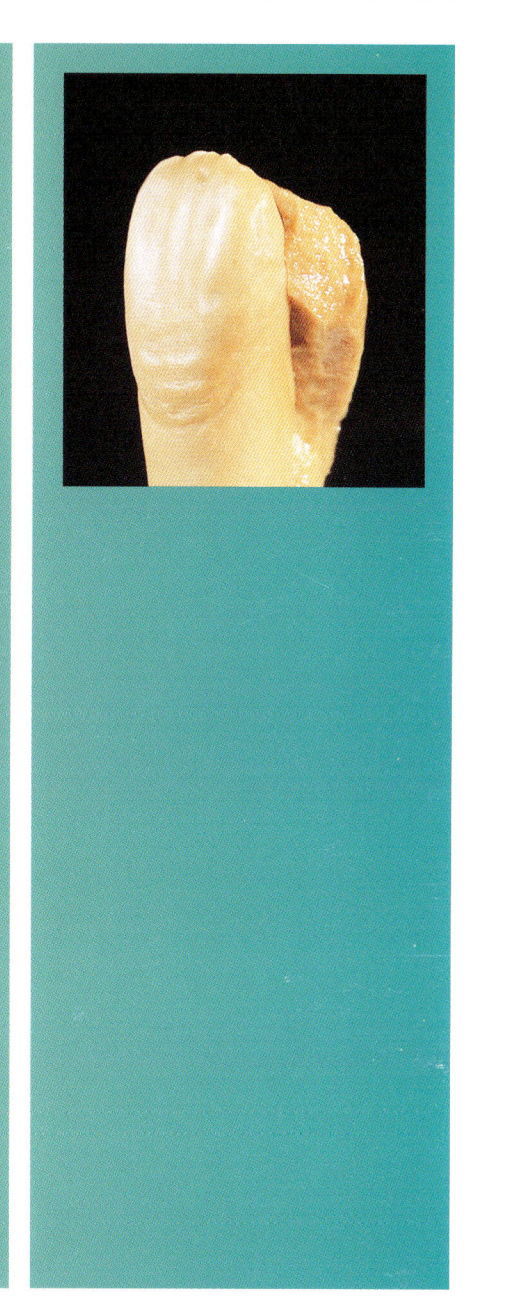

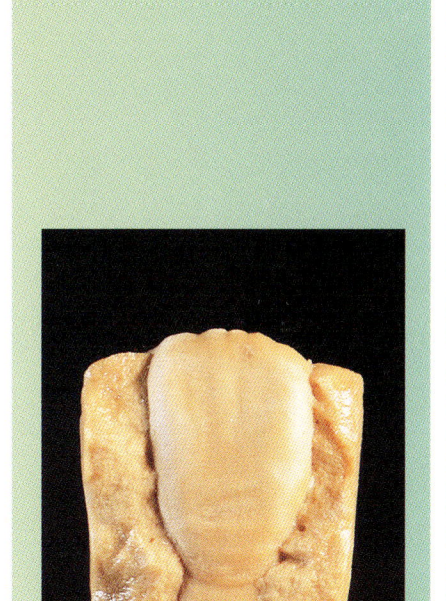

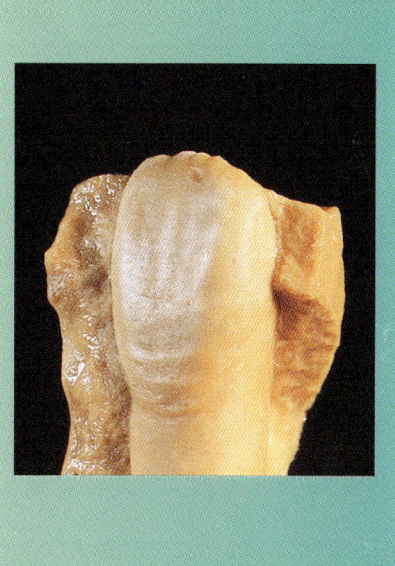

Adjustment of Proximal Contact Areas

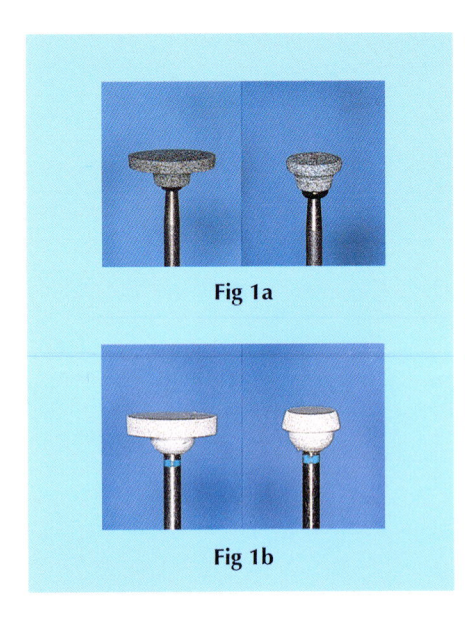

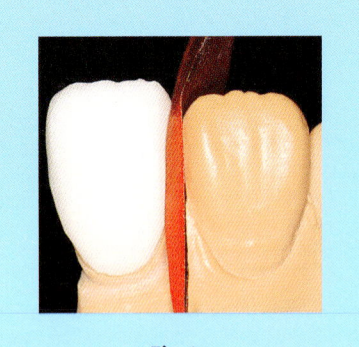

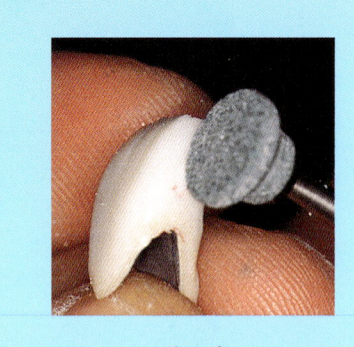

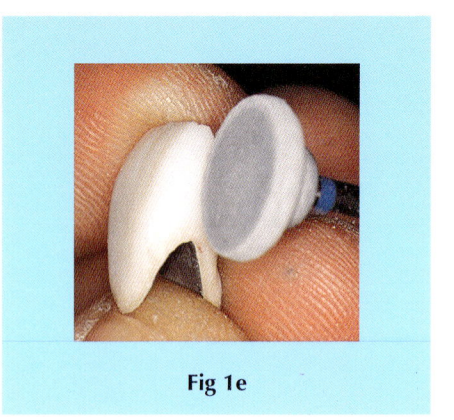

Fig 1a

Fig 1b

Fig 1c

Fig 1d

Fig 1e

Fig 1a Reduce a Shofu Dura Green Stone No. WH6 *(left)* with a Shofu Abrasive Dresser to the desired small size *(right)*.

Fig 1b Reduce a Shofu Ceramiste Soft No. PA *(left)* to the desired small size *(right)*.

Fig 1c Place thin articulating ribbon between the restoration and the adjacent tooth, seat the fired restoration, and check the mark. Since areas other than the contact area may become marked, the proximal contact area must be checked visually before proceeding to the next step.

Fig 1d Adjust the marked area with a Shofu Dura Green Stone No. WH6 (Fig 1a, *right*). Seat the restoration with the articulating ribbon (Fig 1c) and adjust the marked area again. Leave the proximal contact a little tight at this point to allow room for the slight reduction that will take place during polishing. Also, grossly create interproximal space by shaping the proximal transitional surfaces.

Fig 1e After adjusting the surface with the Dura Green Stone, adjust and polish it with a Shofu Ceramiste Soft No. PA (Fig 1b, *right*) to achieve an appropriate proximal contact area.

Fig 1f The crown after adjustment of the mesial and distal proximal contact areas. Labial view *(left)*; incisal view *(right)*.

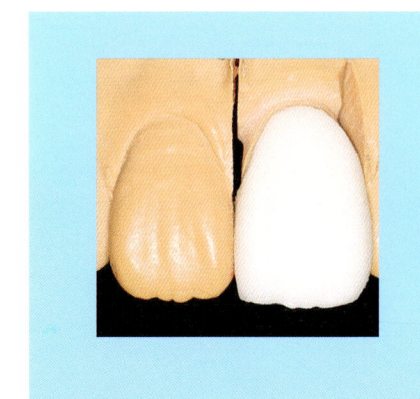

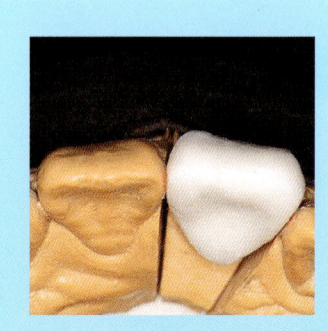

Fig 1f

Figs 1g to 1i Schematic illustrations of possible scenarios in the process of proximal contact point formation.

Fig 1g Proper proximal contact.

Fig 1h Overadjustment of the interproximal space resulted in an open contact.

Fig 1i Proximal contact area is overcontoured and positioned too far labially.

Fig 1g

Fig 1h

Fig 1i

Emphasis

Because the proximal contact area is rather wide, it is necessary to select a starting point. Unless a starting point is selected, the end result may be an open proximal contact (Fig 1h) or improper labial interproximal space (Fig 1i).

The proper mesial proximal contact point of a central incisor is the contact point between the mesial walls of adjacent central incisors in the sagittal plane. Because the reshaping that is done on the mesial dictates the position of the distal proximal point, this contact area will be kept small at this stage.

The reshaping process is started from the mesial side. The proximal contact point is selected as a starting point, then the labial interproximal space is adjusted by opening the proximal transitional surfaces of the mesiolabial marginal ridge to create symmetry with the adjacent tooth.

The proximal contact area should not be left rough after reshaping; it could abrade the stone cast and thus lose the ability to produce an accurate contact area. The roughness would also induce plaque accumulation, because the glazing procedure is not sufficient to eliminate such roughness. Therefore, the proximal contact area should be polished at this stage.

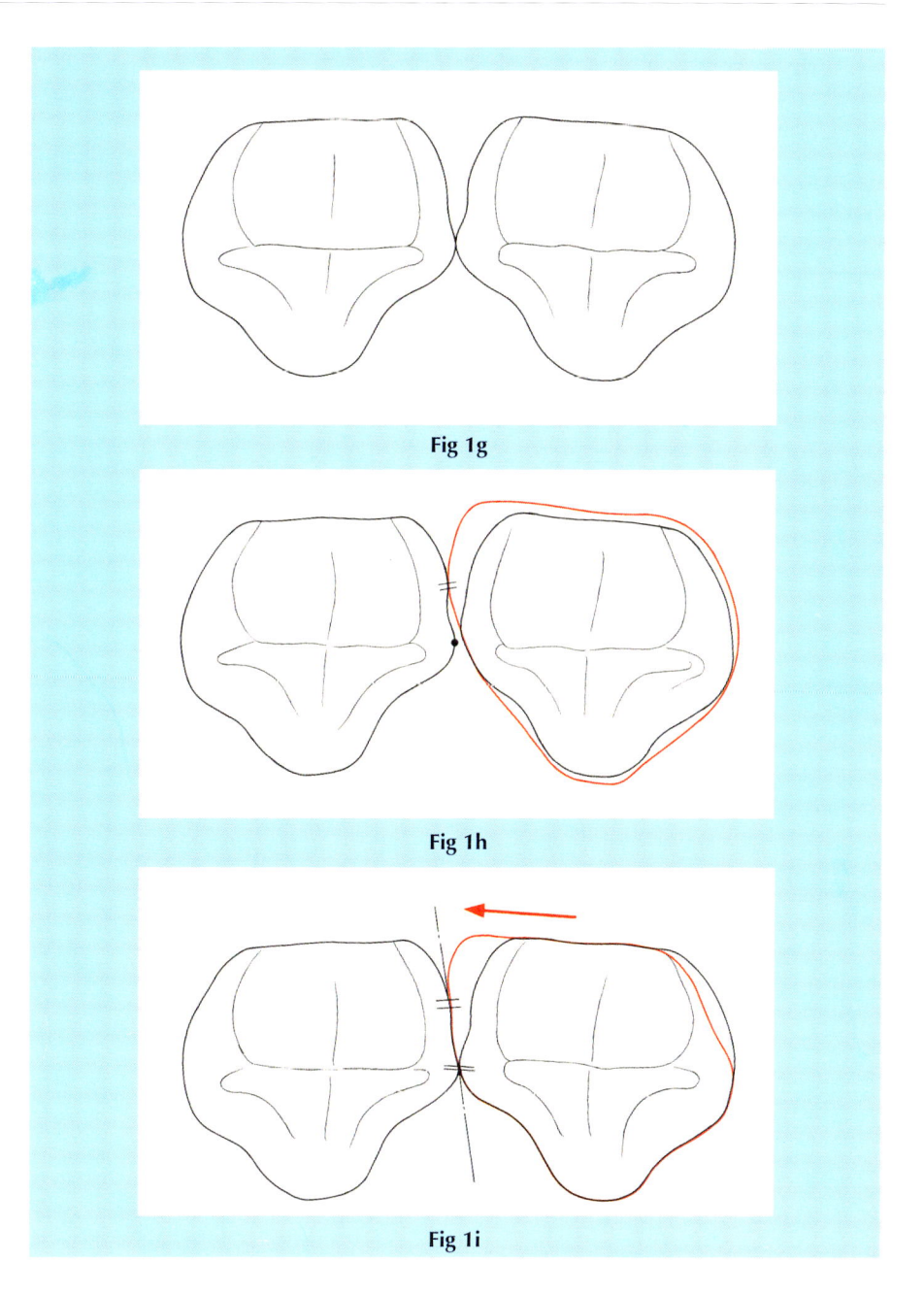

Gross Contouring I: Three-Plane Labial Composition

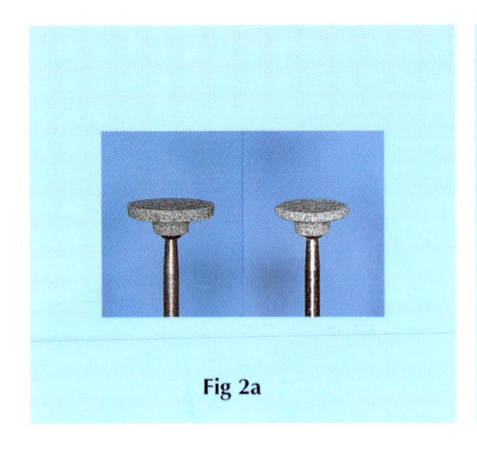

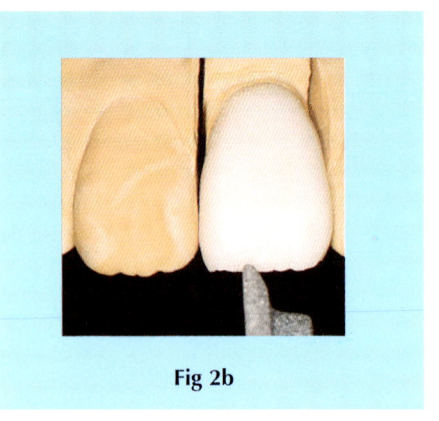

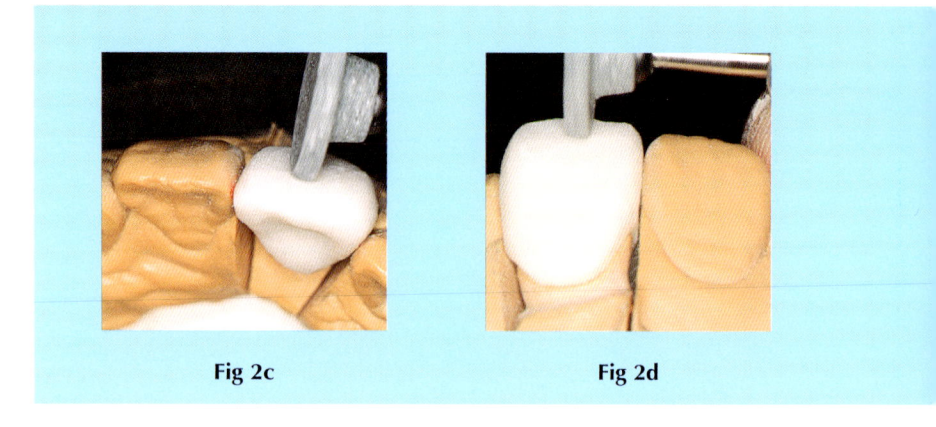

Fig 2a

Fig 2b

Fig 2c

Fig 2d

Fig 2a Modify a Shofu Dura Green Stone No. WH6 *(left)* with a Shofu Abrasive Dresser. Thin the stone in an angle pointing outward, and round the corner *(right)*.

Fig 2b Check and roughly adjust the labiolingual position and length of the incisal edge (labial view). It should be a little longer than the adjacent tooth.

Fig 2c Contour the middle half of the labial surface (incisal view).

Fig 2d Contour the incisal quarter (cervical view).

Fig 2e Contour the cervical quarter and the twist of the crown (labioincisal view).

Fig 2f The restoration after contouring the three-plane labial composition. Labial view *(left)*; incisal view *(center)*; cervical view *(right)*.

Emphasis

After adjustment of the proximal contact areas, the labiolingual position and length of the incisal edge are adjusted from a labial view. This adjustment is typically made according to the occlusal relationship, but the smile line and the occlusal plane can serve as guides if this does not interfere with forming proper occlusal scheme. Adjustments at this stage should be rough and the restoration oversized.

The labial surface is a composition of three planes: the middle half of the labial surface of a natural tooth is relatively long and straight, and the incisal and cervical quarters are inclined lingually, as seen from the proximal view. After the length of the incisal edge has been adjusted, the labial middle half and then the incisal and cervical quarters are shaped. These surfaces are grossly contoured, forming and maintaining the three-plane labial composition. At this stage, use the modified Shofu Dura Green Stone No. WH6 as shown in Fig 2a.

During the contouring procedure, it is important to check the shape of the restoration from various angles as shown in Fig 2f. The working cast is rotated to different viewing angles, and the arch formed by the incisal line of both central incisors is used as a guide to adjust the three-plane labial composition to make a rough symmetric shape similar to that of the adjacent central incisor.

Fig 2e

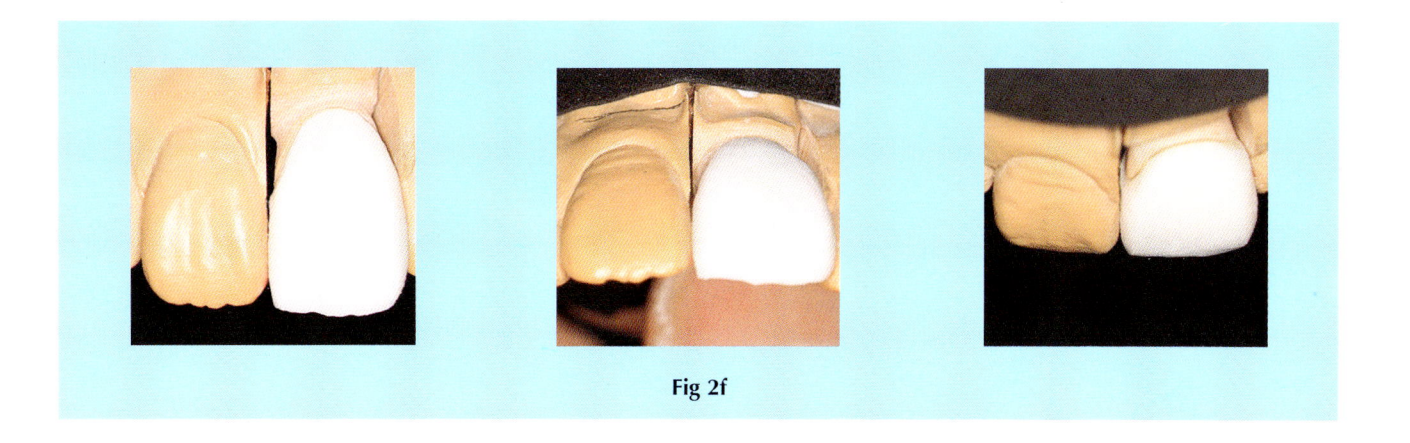

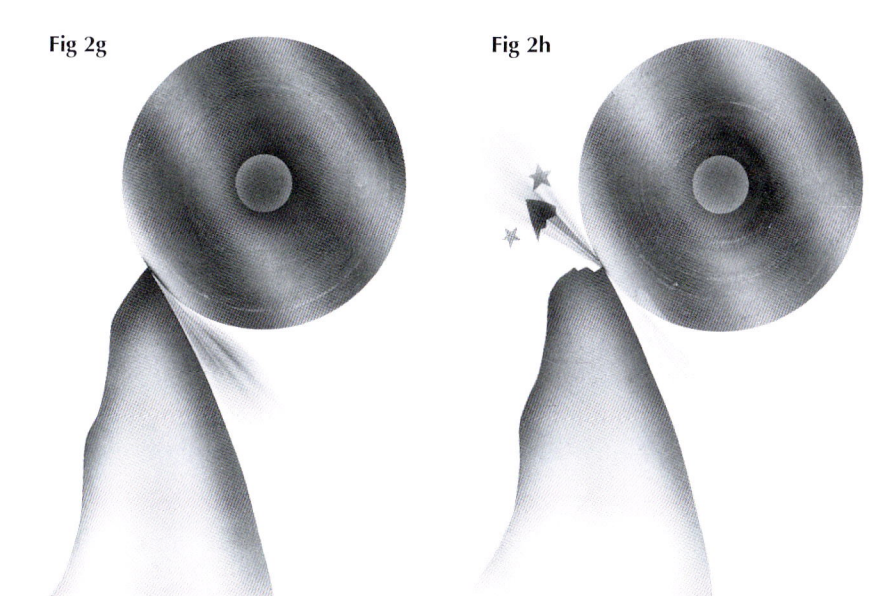

Fig 2f

Figs 2g and 2h The direction of rotation of the disk is important to avoid chipping of the porcelain.

Fig 2g Proper direction of rotation.

Fig 2h Wrong direction of rotation.

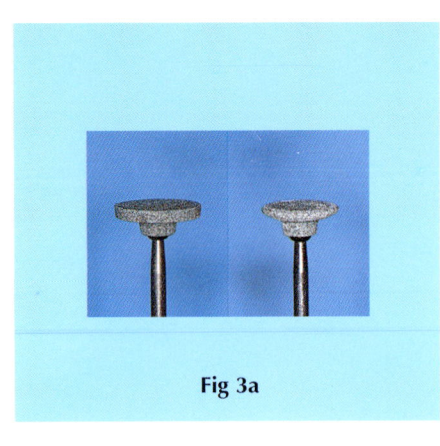

Gross Contouring II: Marginal Ridges and Proximal Transitional Surfaces

Fig 3a

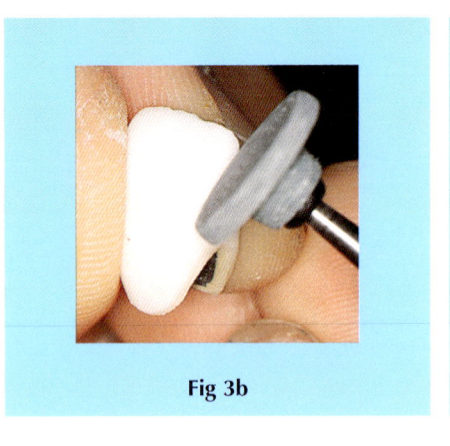

Fig 3b

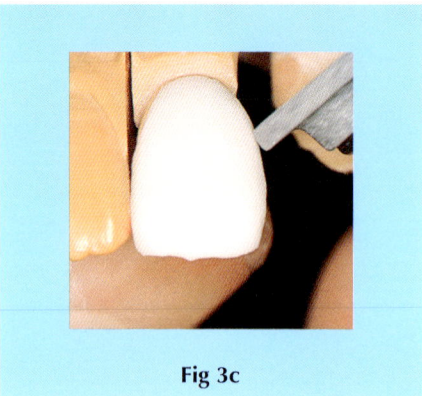

Fig 3c

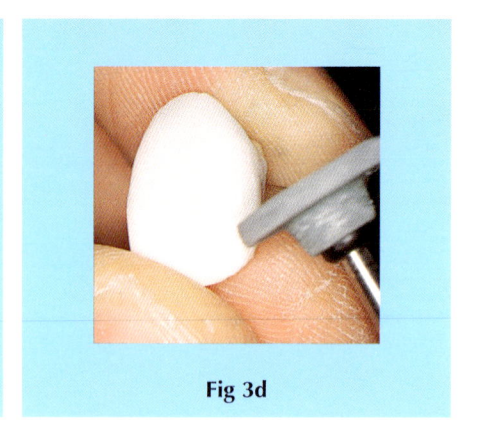

Fig 3d

Fig 3a Modify a Shofu Dura Green Stone No. WH6 *(left)* with a Shofu Abrasive Dresser. Thin the stone in an angle pointing outward, and round the corner *(right)*.

Fig 3b Adjust the mesial marginal ridge and the mesial proximal transitional surface. Since the mesial side serves as the reference for the width of the tooth crown and the shape of the distal side, complete the mesial aspect meticulously prior to working on the distal side.

Fig 3c Adjust the distal marginal ridge and the distal proximal transitional surface on the working cast.

Fig 3d Remove the restoration from the working cast to contour the area of the distal proximal transitional surface that cannot be contoured while the restoration is on the cast.

Fig 3e Remove the crown from the working cast, and evaluate the width and the overall shape.

Fig 3f The crown after contouring of the marginal ridges and the proximal transitional surfaces (labial view).

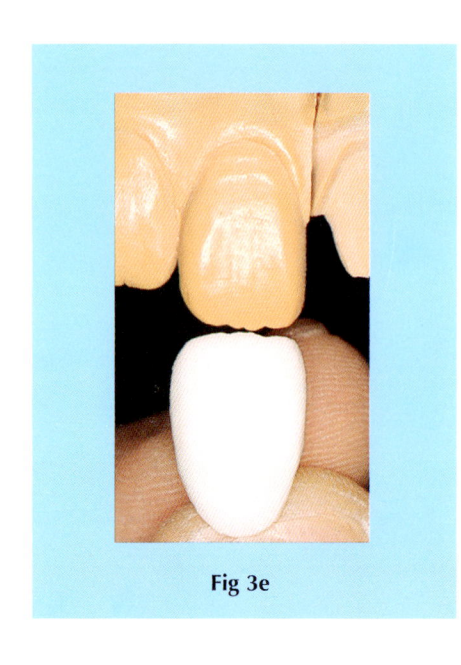

Fig 3e

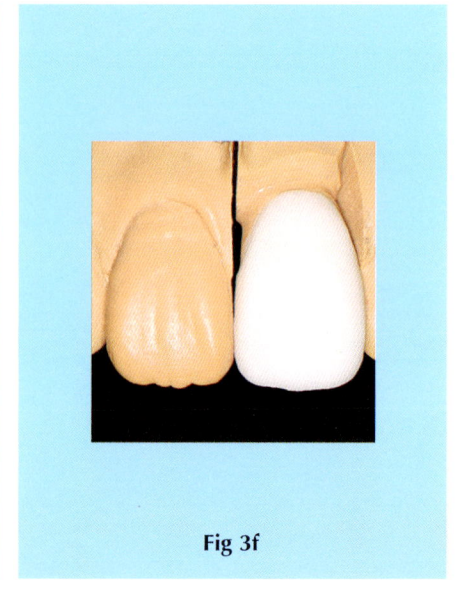

Fig 3f

Fig 3g Chart of proximal transitional surface. Labial view *(top)*; incisal view *(bottom)*.

Emphasis

The width of the surface from the peak, or height of contour, of the marginal ridge to the proximal contact point is the proximal transitional surface, and its size varies from tooth to tooth. In the particular tooth presented in Fig 3g, the width of the proximal transitional surface is narrow in the incisal area, wider toward the middle of the tooth crown, and then narrow again in the cervical area.

Contouring of the mesial proximal transitional surfaces should be completed meticulously prior to adjusting the distal surface. This is necessary because the mesial proximal transitional surface and the mesial marginal ridge will serve as the references for the distance to the distal marginal ridge and the distal proximal transitional surface, as well as the width of the tooth crown. The adjusted crown should be oversized at this stage to allow for shrinkage.

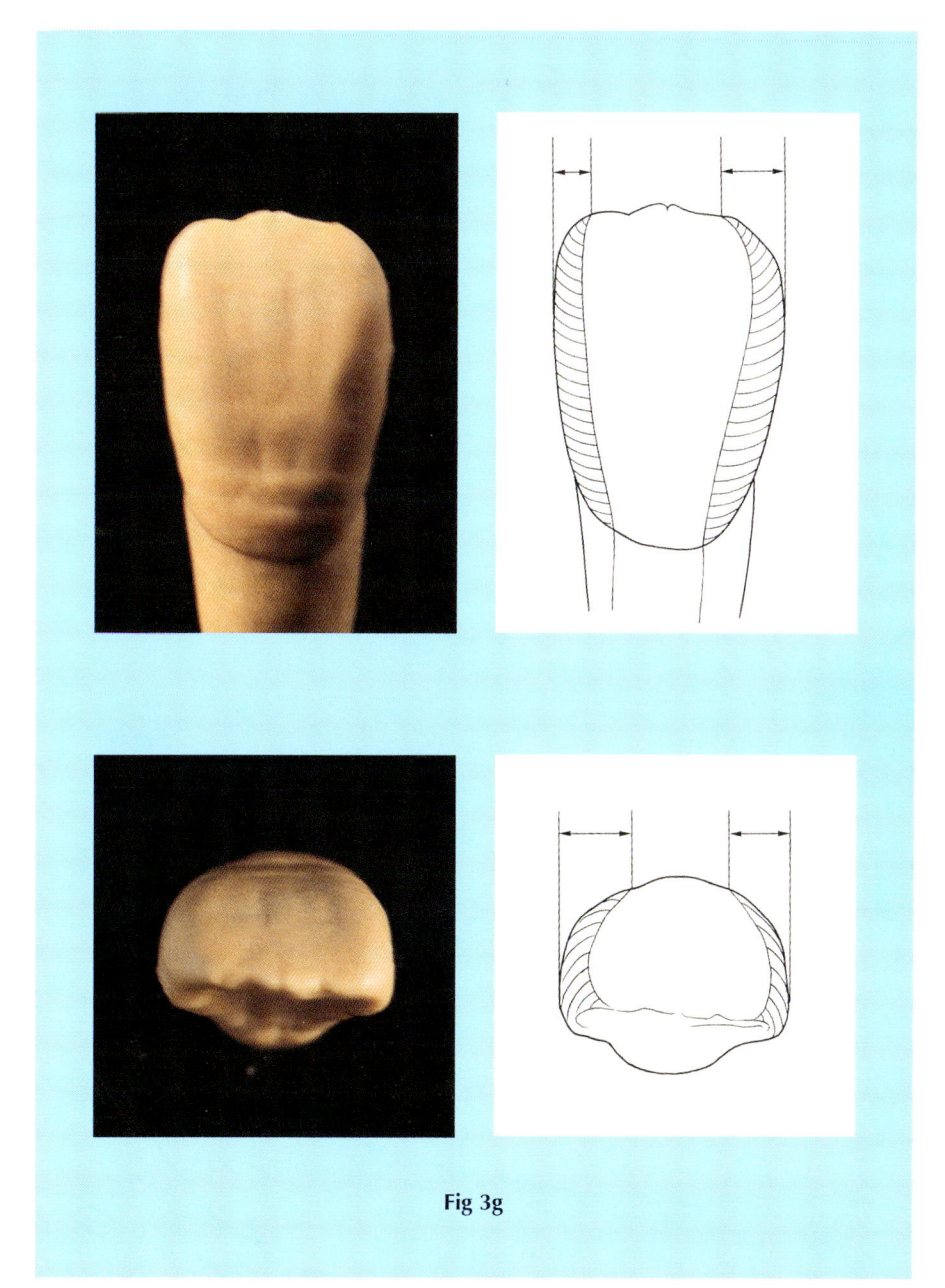

Fig 3g

Gross Contouring III: Lingual Surface

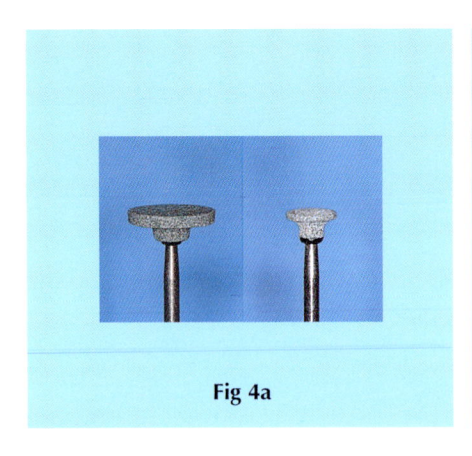

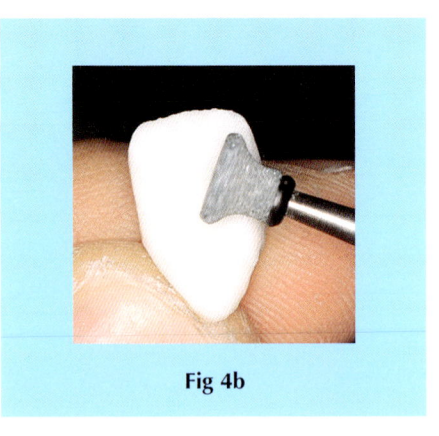

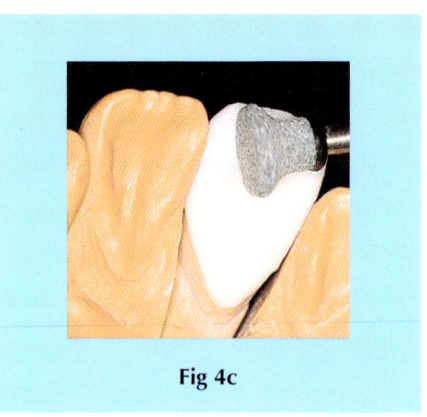

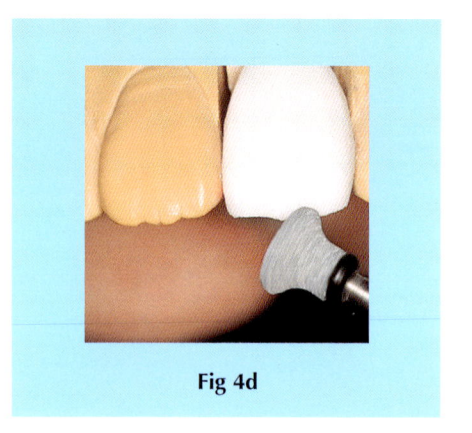

Fig 4a

Fig 4b

Fig 4c

Fig 4d

Fig 4a Further reduce the Shofu Dura Green Stone No. WH6 *(left)*, to make it even smaller *(right)*.

Fig 4b Adjust the height of both the mesial and distal marginal ridges using the contralateral tooth on the working cast as a guide to form symmetry between the teeth. Next, roughly contour the lingual fossa and the lingual grooves on the working cast.

Fig 4c Contour the escape routes of the lingual fossa to the proximal surface and the continuity of the lingual marginal ridge to the incisal edge.

Fig 4d Contour the incisal edge with consideration to its relationship to the lingual side (labial view).

Fig 4e Ceramic restoration after adjustment of the lingual side. It is oversized at this stage. Lingual view *(left)*; incisal view *(right)*.

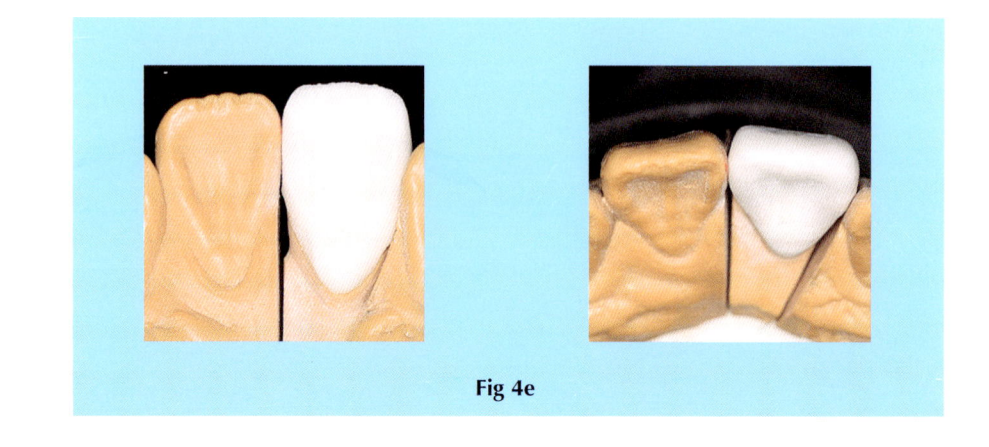

Fig 4e

Fig 4f Stone model demonstrating the escape routes of the lingual fossa and the continuity of the ridges.

Fig 4g Schematic illustrations of the escape routes of the lingual fossa and the continuity of the ridges. Correct *(left)*; incorrect *(right)*.

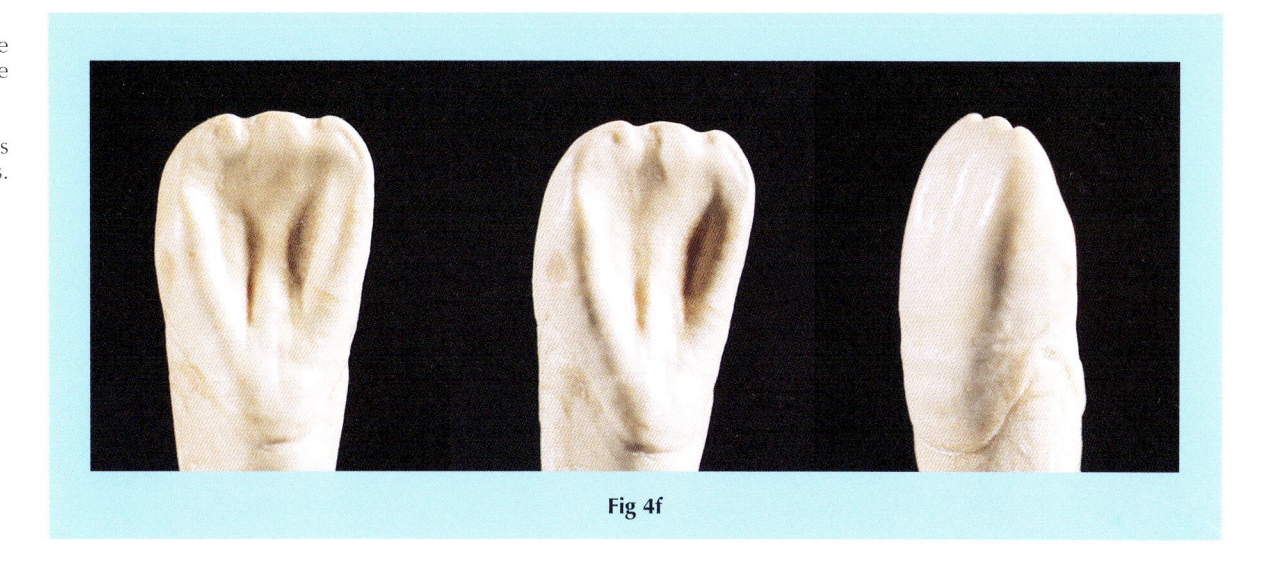

Fig 4f

Emphasis

The lingual marginal ridges usually do not extend to the incisal edge and therefore create the escape routes of the lingual fossa toward the proximal surface. However, careful observation reveals that the lingual marginal ridge, which meets the peak of the labial marginal ridge and continues to the incisal ridge, surrounds the lingual fossa. The shape is very different between the mesial and distal sides, as indicated in chapter 2 in the discussion of the continuity of each surface form.

Accurate contouring of the lingual fossa escape routes and continuous ridges reproduces the characteristic three-dimensional appearance of the lingual aspect of the incisal edge in labial-lateral or lateral view.

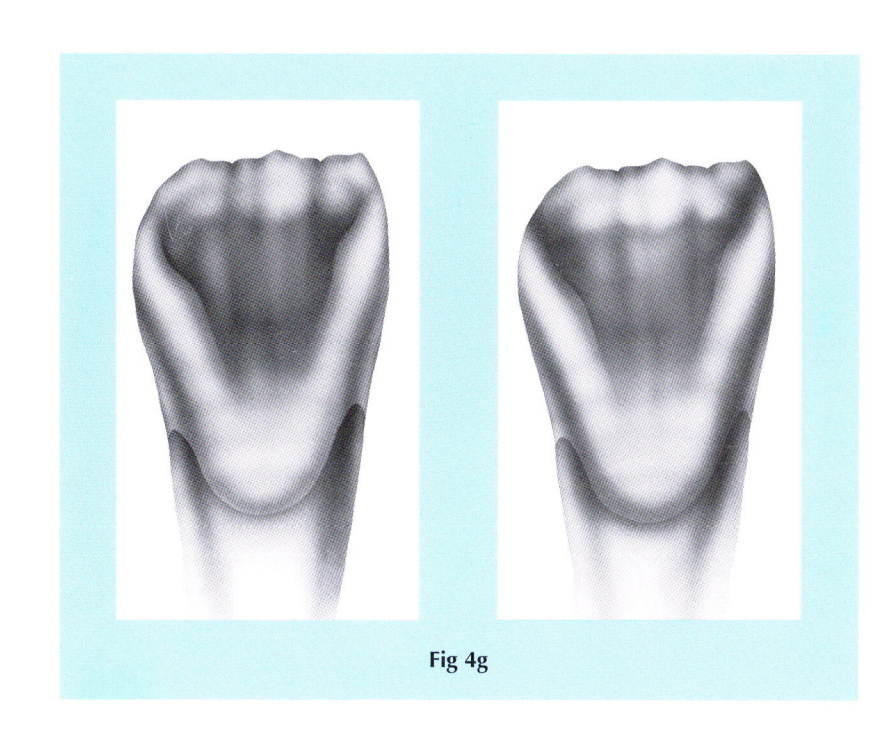

Fig 4g

Intermediate Finishing I: Line Angles, Transitional Areas, and Primary Ridges

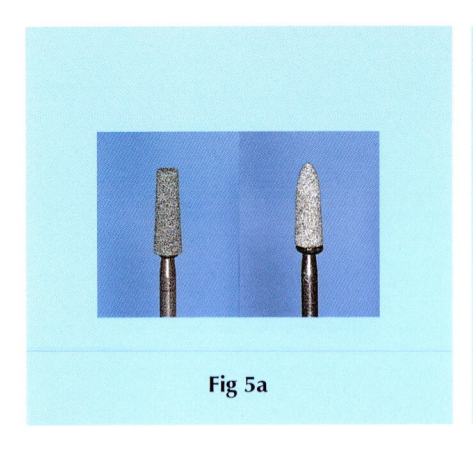

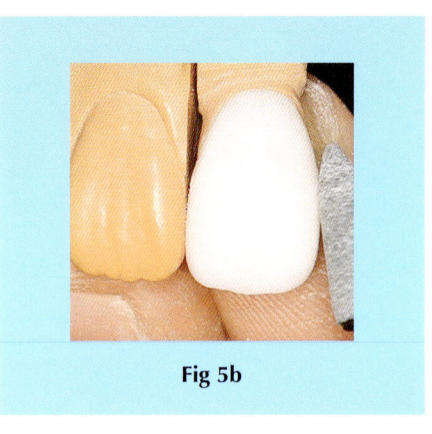

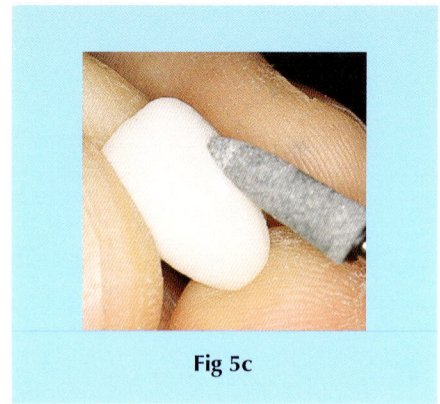

Fig 5a Modify a Shofu Dura Green Stone No. TC4 *(left)* to a bullet shape *(right)* with a Shofu Abrasive Dresser.

Fig 5b Evaluate the ceramic restoration on the working cast (labial view).

Fig 5c The area that cannot be contoured with the restoration on the working cast is contoured off the cast.

Fig 5d Modify a Shofu Dura Green Stone No. TC4 *(left)* to an angle *(right)* with a Shofu Abrasive Dresser.

Fig 5e Contour the labial grooves to the same depth as the contralateral tooth (incisal view).

Fig 5f Contour the marginal ridges and the central ridge to form symmetry with the contralateral tooth. Evaluate from the labial view.

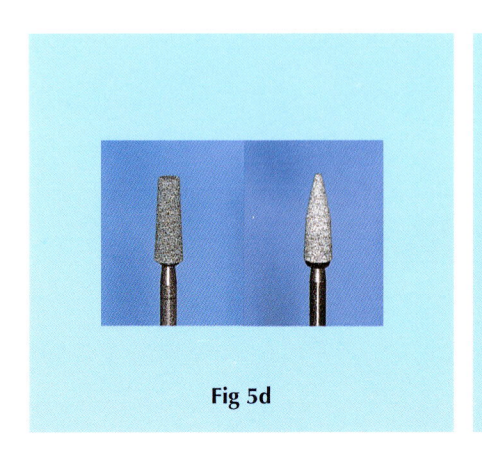

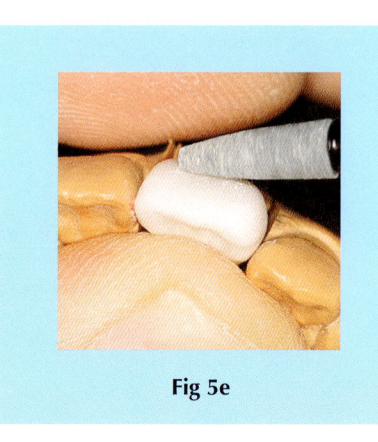

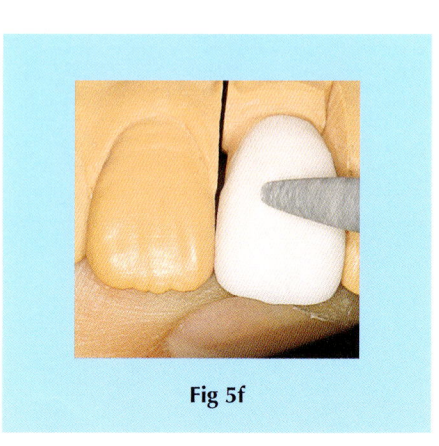

Fig 5g

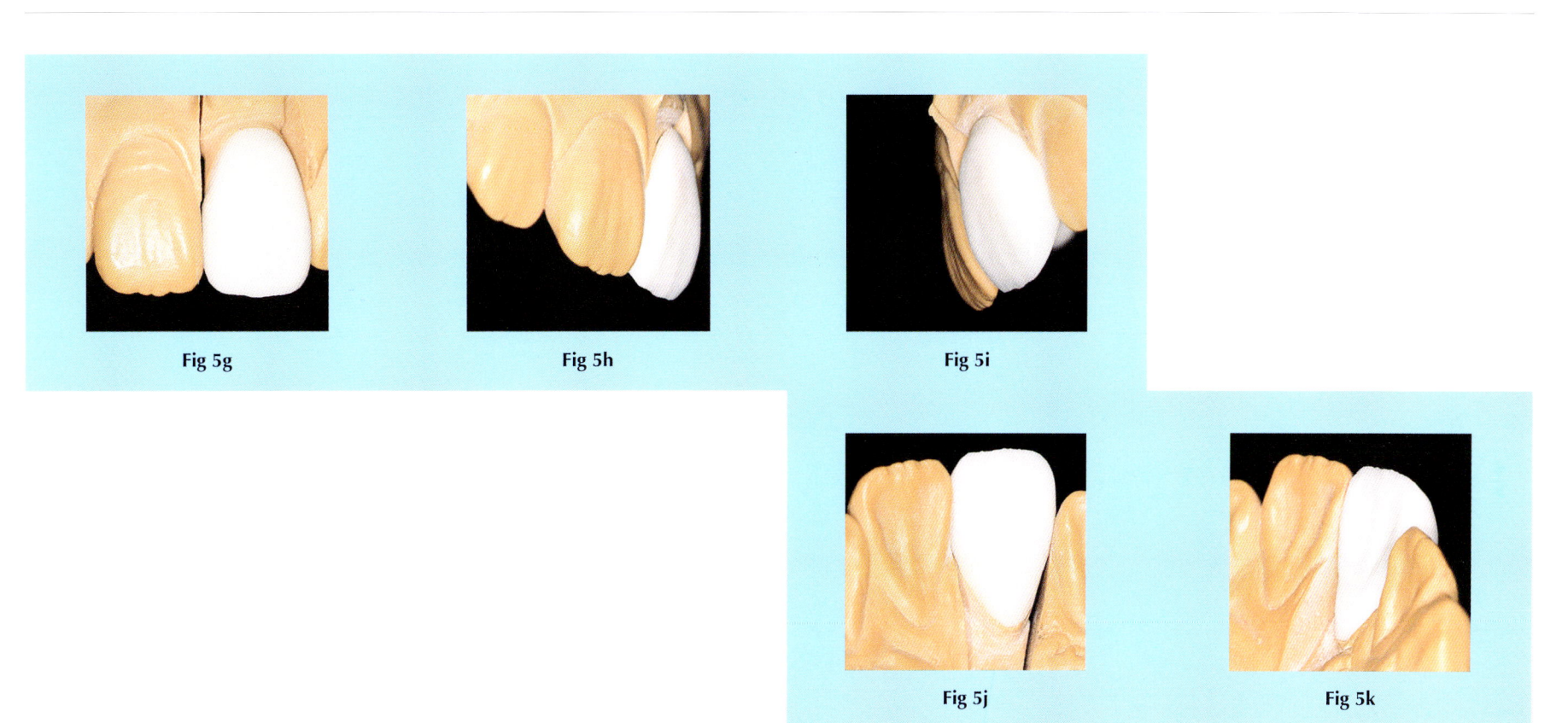

Fig 5h

Fig 5i

Fig 5j

Fig 5k

Emphasis

In the gross contouring stage, the line angles are sharper than those of the contralateral side. In this second stage, the roundness of the line angles of the contralateral side is carefully examined and reproduced into the ceramic restoration. The mesio and disto-incisal line angles are contoured accordingly. Use the bullet-shaped Shofu Dura Green Stone No. TC4 for this stage of finishing.

Finally, labial and lingual grooves and ridges are roughly contoured using the angled Shofu Dura Green Stone No. TC4 shown in Fig 5d.

Figs 5g to 5k The ceramic restoration after intermediate finishing (contouring of the incisal line angles and the main ridges).

Fig 5g Labial view.

Fig 5h Mesial-lateral view.

Fig 5i Distal-lateral view.

Fig 5j Lingual view.

Fig 5k Distal-lateral view.

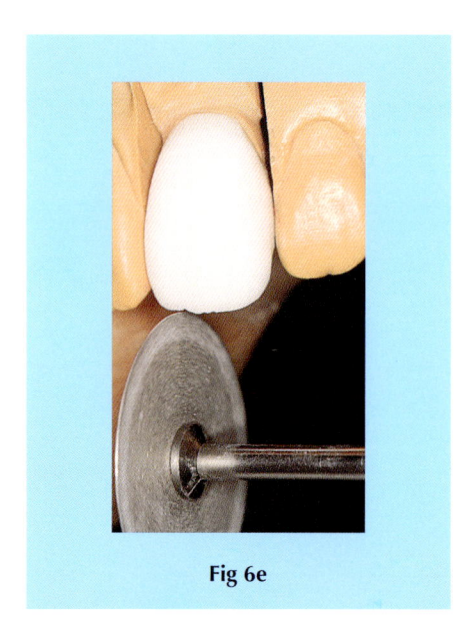

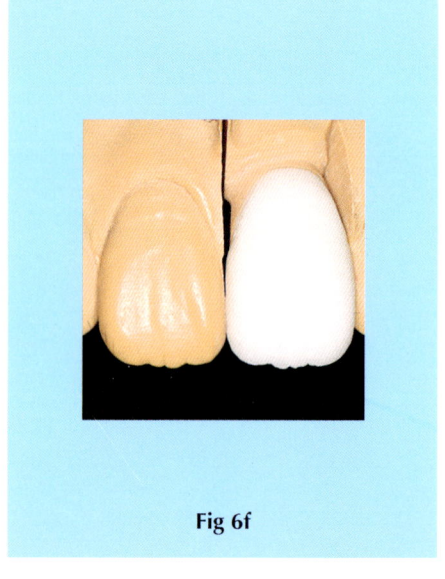

Intermediate Finishing II: Transverse Ridges and Grooves

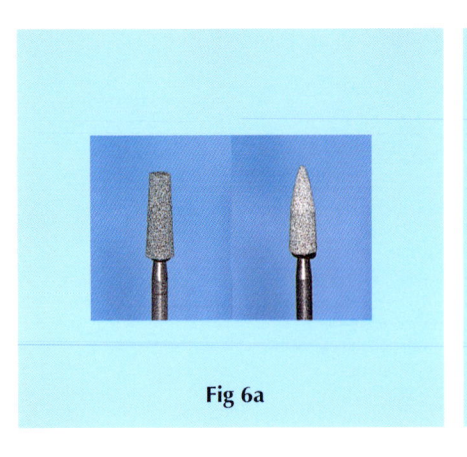

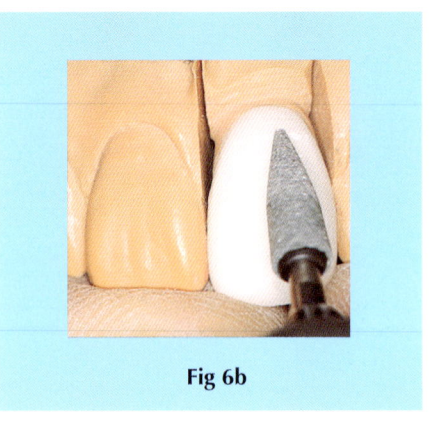

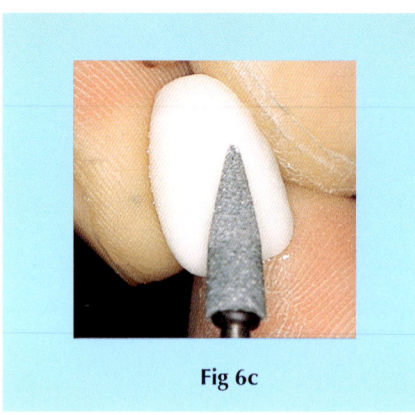

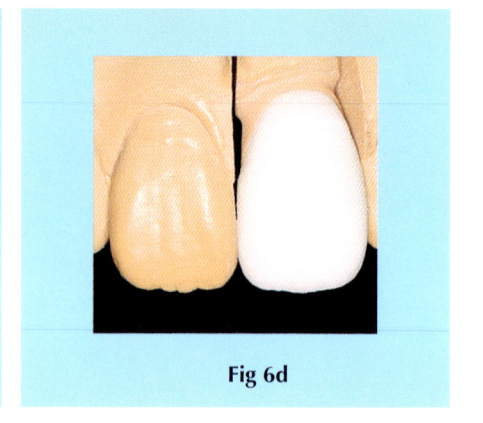

Fig 6a

Fig 6b

Fig 6c

Fig 6d

Fig 6a Modify a Shofu Dura Green Stone No. TC4 *(left)* to an angle *(right)*, as was done in Fig 5d.

Fig 6b Contour the transverse grooves on the working cast to form symmetry with the contralateral tooth.

Fig 6c Contour the transverse ridges, smoothing off the transverse grooves, which were formed in Fig 6b. Extend the ridge to the proximal surface.

Fig 6d Ceramic restoration after contouring of the transverse ridges (labial view).

Fig 6e Contour developmental grooves at the incisal edge with a diamond disk (Shofu Summa Disk S61UT, 19-mm diameter, 0.15-mm thickness), and contour the incisal aspect of the developmental lobes.

Fig 6f Ceramic restoration after contouring of the transverse ridges and incisal aspect of the developmental lobes (labial view).

Fig 6e

Fig 6f

Figs 6g to 6i Schematic illustrations of the transverse ridges and grooves.

Fig 6g Proper shaping of transverse ridges and grooves.

Fig 6h Improper shaping. Transverse ridges and grooves are too straight.

Fig 6i Improper shaping. Transverse ridges and grooves are crossing each other.

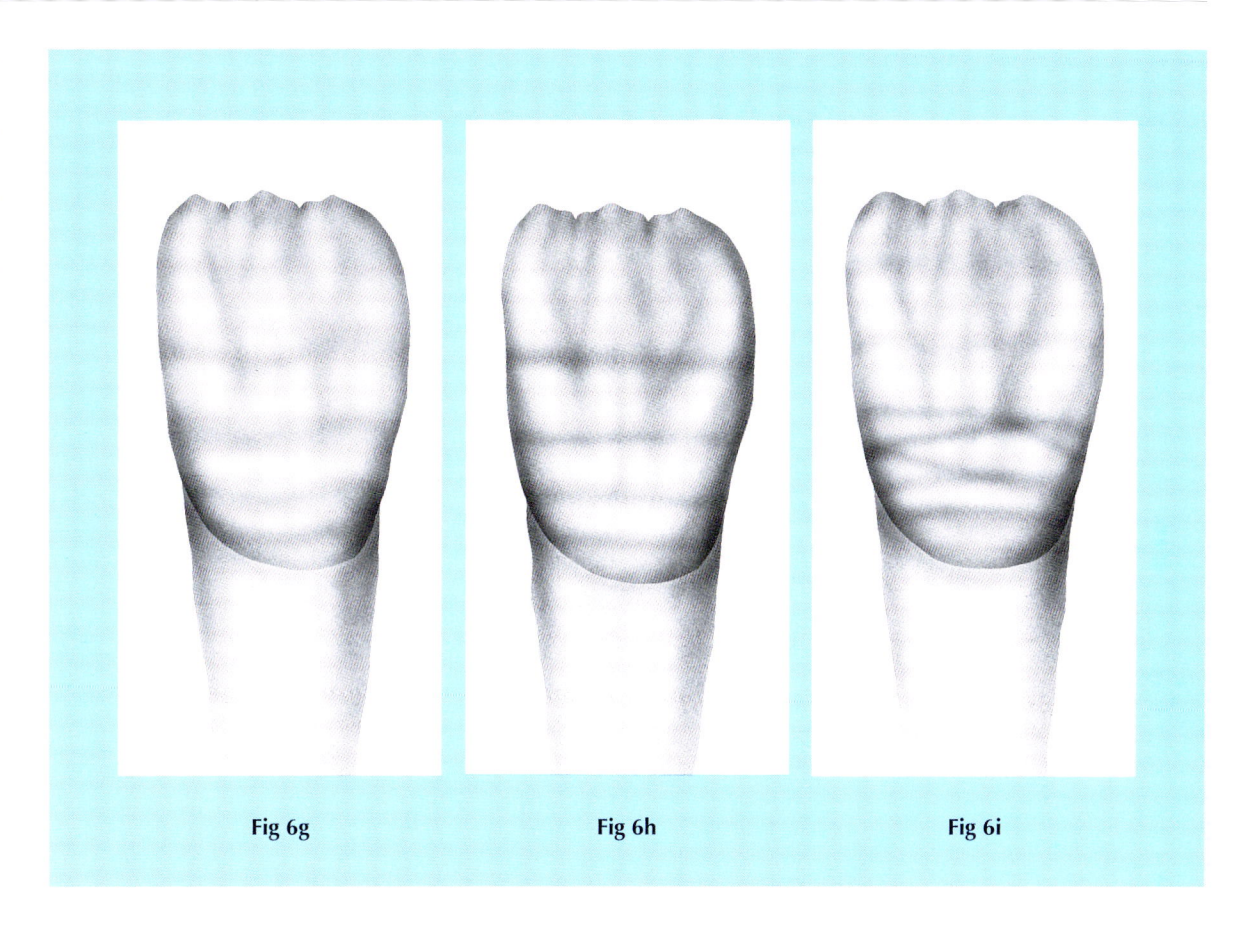

Fig 6g   **Fig 6h**   **Fig 6i**

Emphasis

Trying to form the labial and transverse grooves during contouring is a common mistake. Instead, it is important to create ridges, such as marginal ridges, central ridges, or transverse ridges. As a result, these will form the labial or transverse grooves.

The width and/or the location of the transverse ridges should be carefully considered. The transverse ridges run at right angles to the long axis of the tooth and should be parallel to each other. Transverse ridges never cross each other or present a mesiodistal difference in spacing between each ridge.

At this stage, developmental lobes and grooves are contoured at the incisal edge. The characteristics of the contralateral tooth, such as wear facets, should be observed and reproduced according to the patient's age.

Use a rather thinly contoured Shofu Dura Green Stone No. TC4 (Fig 6a) to reproduce transverse ridges and a diamond disk (Shofu Summa Disk S61UT, 19-mm diameter, 0.15-mm thickness) to form the incisal aspect of the developmental lobes.

Finishing I: Gross Surface Texture

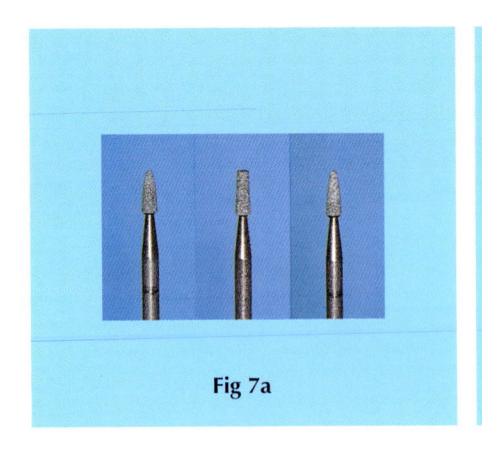

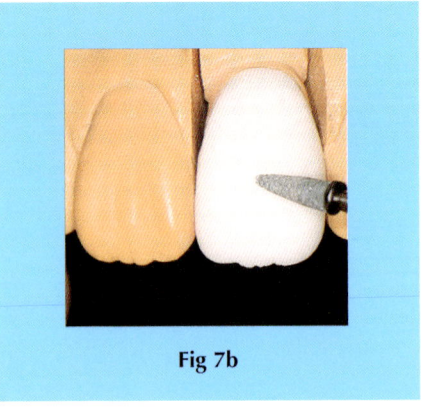

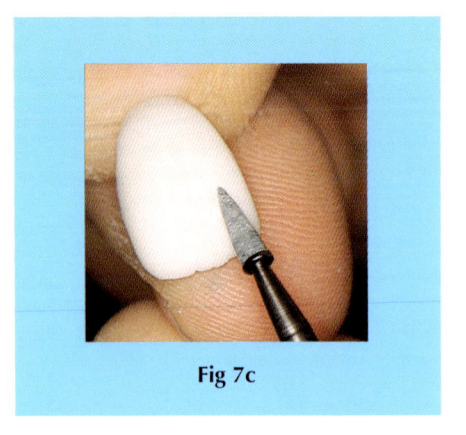

Fig 7a

Fig 7b

Fig 7c

Fig 7a Use a thin, cone-shaped *(left)* Shofu Dura Green Stone No. TC1 *(center)* and its angled version *(right)*.

Fig 7b To form symmetry with the contralateral tooth, use the tip of the angle-modified Dura Green Stone (Fig 7a, *right*) to contour a labial groove. Complete this step with the restoration on the working cast.

Fig 7c With the restoration off the working cast, smooth the marginal and central ridges and make them more prominent using the Dura Green Stone shown in Fig 7a *(left)*.

Fig 7d Ceramic restoration with properly contoured ridges. Labial view *(left)*; mesial-lateral view *(right)*.

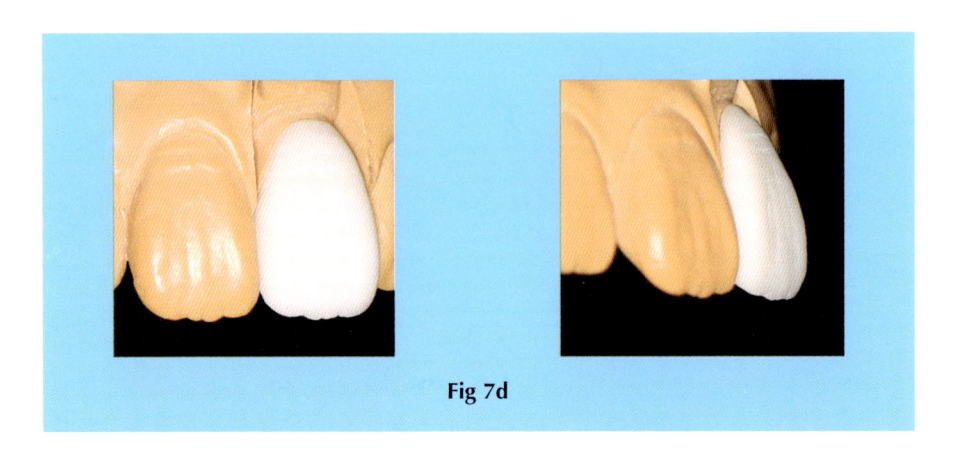

Emphasis

At this point, the thickness and the direction of the main ridges and the transverse ridges are not finalized, and the surface is rough due to the coarse grinding instruments. Therefore, finer points are recommended to smooth the surface of the ceramic restoration and to recontour and smooth the main ridges and the transverse ridges. Smoothing and recontouring result in better light reflection from the labial ridges and thus a natural-looking restoration.

In addition to the recontouring of these ridges, more detailed surface characteristics, such as accessory ridges, V-shaped grooves, and proximal grooves, should be formed at this stage.

Use thinned modifications of the Shofu Dura Green Stone No. TC1 (Fig 7a) for this procedure.

Fig 7d

Fig 7e

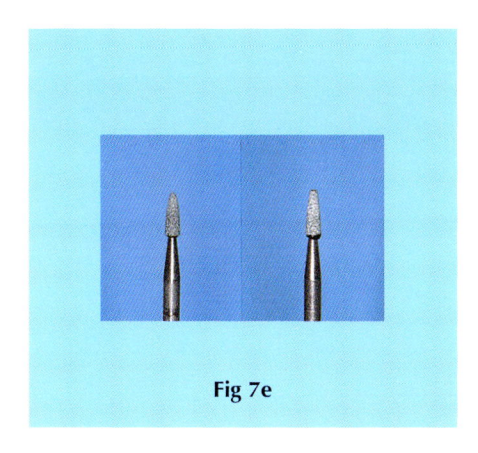

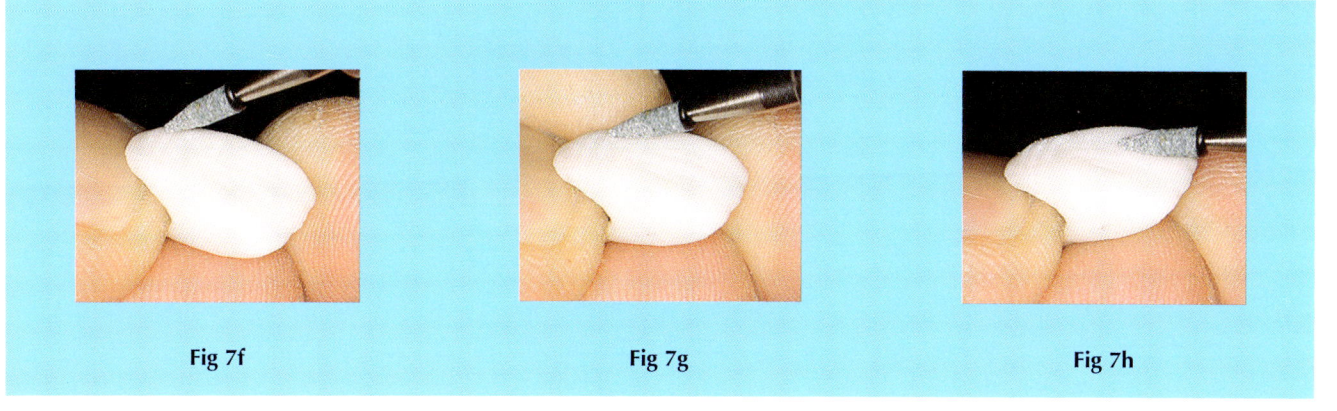

Fig 7f

Fig 7g

Fig 7h

Emphasis

The depth of the transverse grooves varies according to the location of the groove on the tooth. They are deep from the incisal edge to the middle and shallow toward the cervical area. Tilting the Dura Green Stone appropriately will reproduce the sagittal shape of the transverse grooves.

A modified Dura Green Stone No. TC1 with a flattened tip is recommended to form transverse grooves. As shown in Fig 7f, the stone is angled against the surface to form a narrow transverse groove. The transverse groove in Fig 7g is located incisally to the groove in Fig 7f, and the point should be less angled to form a deeper and wider groove. The transverse groove in Fig 7h, is located incisally to the groove in Fig 7g, and the point is even less angled to form a shallow and rather wide groove.

Transverse grooves are less distinct when they intersect longitudinal ridges and more distinct when they intersect longitudinal grooves.

Fig 7e Modify a Shofu Dura Green Stone No. TC1 slightly wider than the one shown in Fig 7a *(left)* and flatten its tip *(right)*.

Figs 7f to 7h Hold the instrument at different angles according to the location of the transverse groove.

Fig 7i Schematic illustration showing various positions of the instrument according to the location of the transverse grooves.

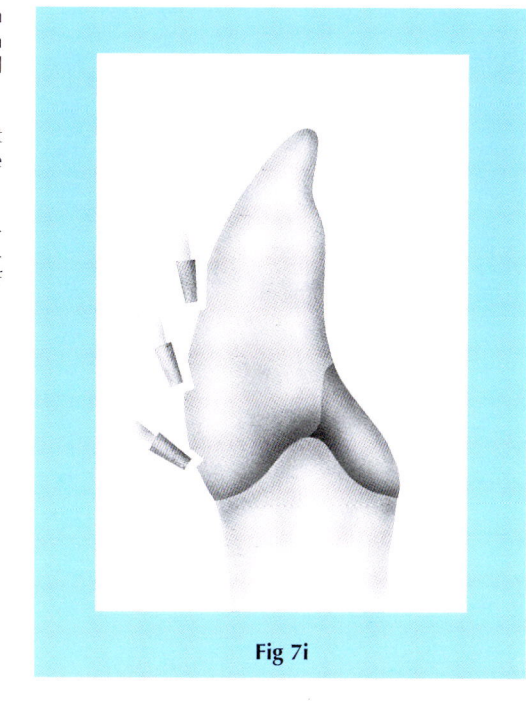

Fig 7i

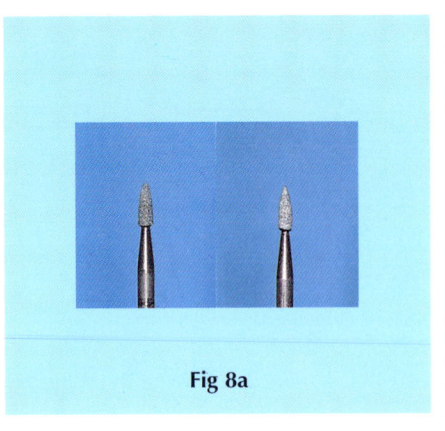

Finishing II: Detailed Surface Texture and Polishing

Fig 8a

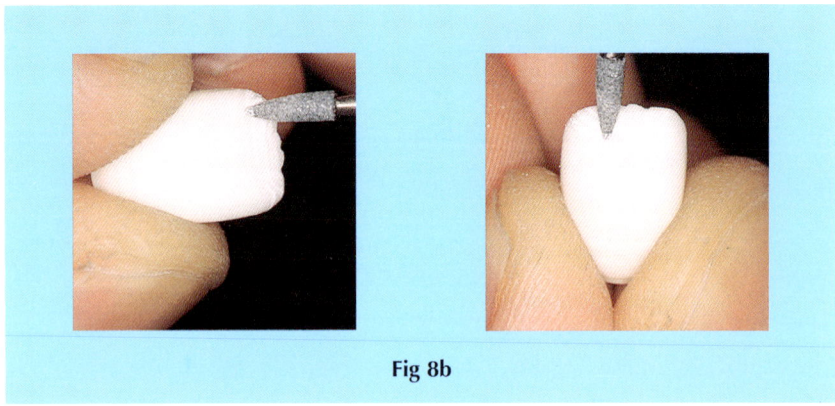

Fig 8b

Contouring of perikymata

Fig 8a Modify a Shofu Dura Green Stone No. TC1 *(left)* with a Shofu Abrasive Dresser to a bullet shape *(right)*.

Fig 8b Contouring of perikymata. The bullet-shaped Dura Green Stone is moved in a mesiodistal direction to form a circle. The tip of the middle labial developmental lobe is the imaginary center of this circle. If the instrument is angled rather than pointed, it will form a perikymata that is too distinct. Start from the distal side *(left)* and slide the point in a circular motion toward the mesial side *(right)*.

Fig 8c The crown after contouring of perikymata. Labial view *(left)*; mesial-lateral view *(center)*; incisal view *(right)*.

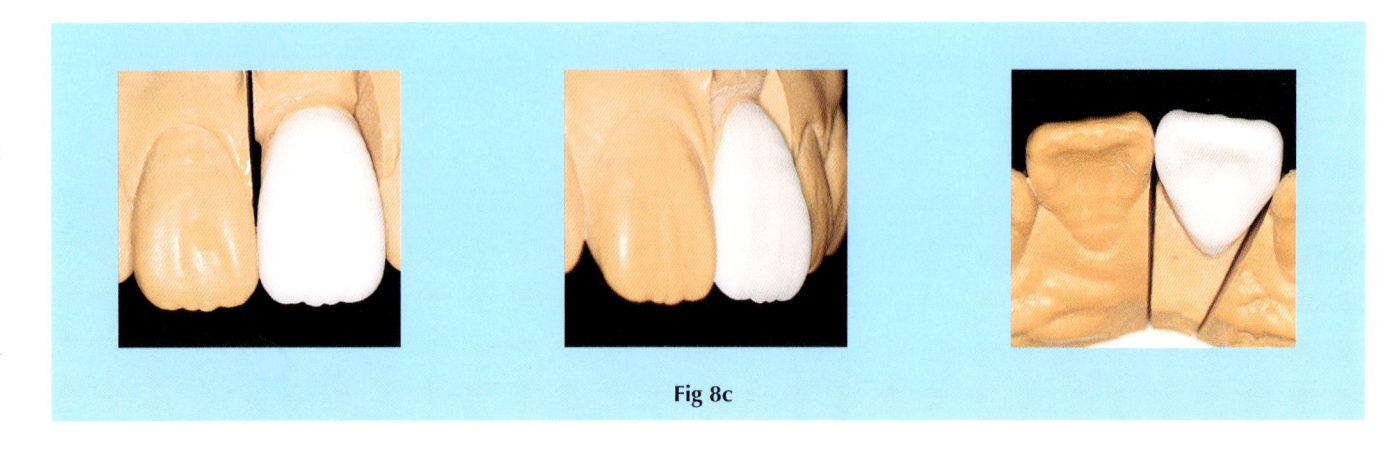

Fig 8c

Final contouring

Figs 9a to 9c Use a Shofu Robot Carbide Cutter No. SH33 to finalize the incisal aspect of developmental lobes and developmental grooves. In addition to contouring the labial side, also contour the lingual side to reproduce the continuity of the developmental grooves from the labial to the lingual.

Fig 9a Contouring from the labial side.

Fig 9b Contouring from the lingual side.

Fig 9c Contouring of the scaly surface of the cervical area. Move the pointed instrument seen in Fig 8a in a mesiodistal direction intermittently.

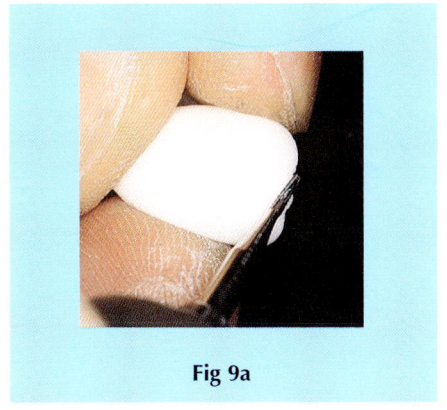

Fig 9a

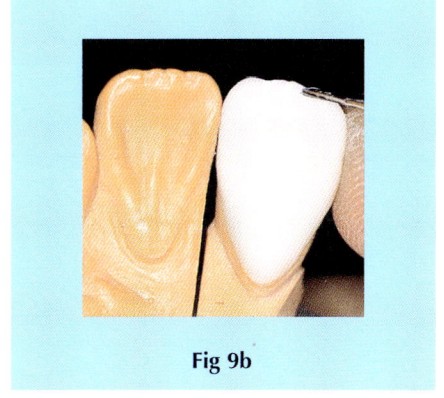

Fig 9b

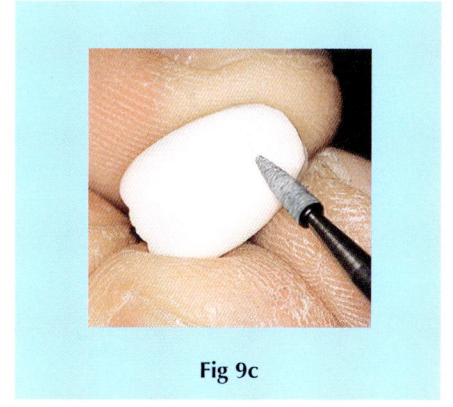

Fig 9c

Emphasis

In this final stage, the more detailed surface texture and the smooth, shiny surface that are characteristic of abrasion or attrition are created.

A typical surface detail is perikymata. Because perikymata are very subtle grooves, they disappear in areas prone to abrasion, but they remain for many years in the areas of the labial grooves or the proximal surfaces. These differences in smoothness give the tooth a natural appearance. Polishing can reproduce this effect.

Canines often have a small, scaly, rugged surface at the cervical area. The tooth with distinct developmental lobes at the incisal area, as shown here, usually has distinct developmental grooves, incisal slope, incisal ridge, and incisal groove. These characteristics are also formed at this final stage.

Surface polishing

Fig 10a Use a modified Shofu Ceramiste Soft No. PB *(right)* for polishing.

Fig 10b Use the tip of the modified Shofu Ceramiste Soft No. PB to eliminate any scratches from previous contouring and create a smooth, shiny labial surface.

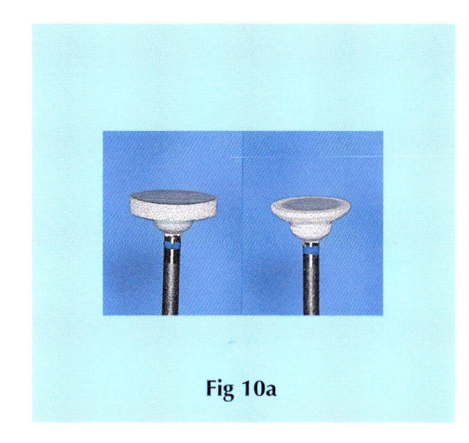

Fig 10a

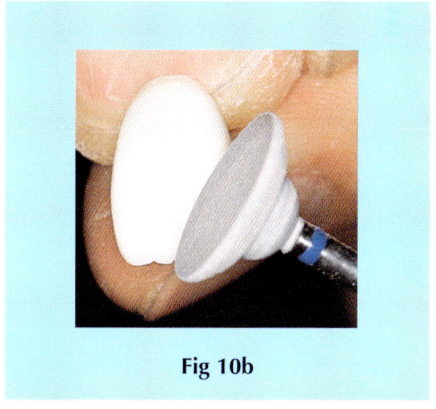

Fig 10b

Completion

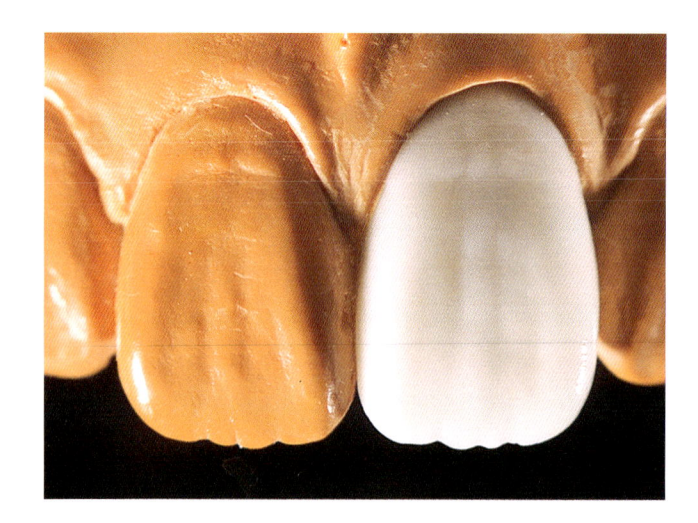

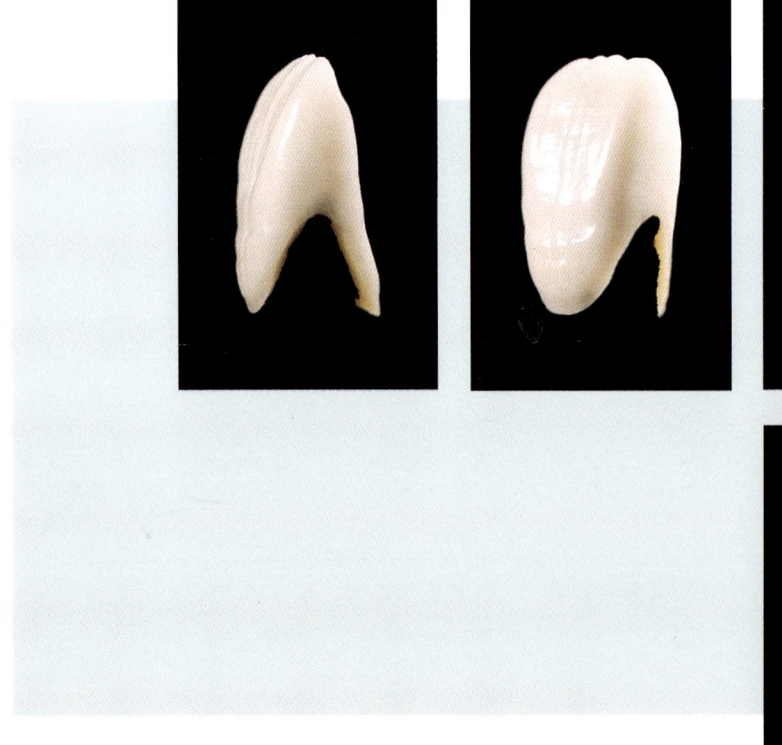

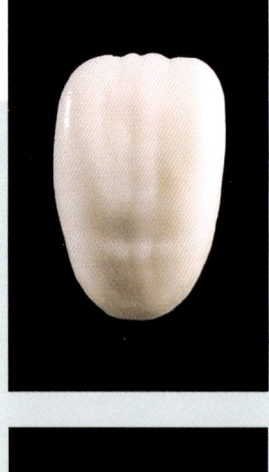

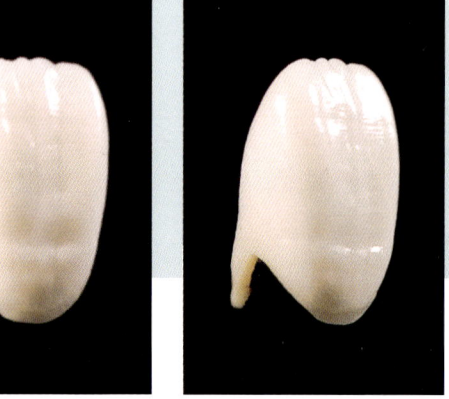

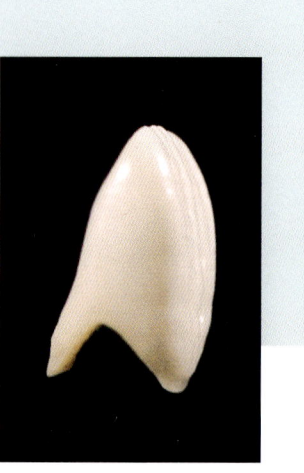

ch 4 | 75

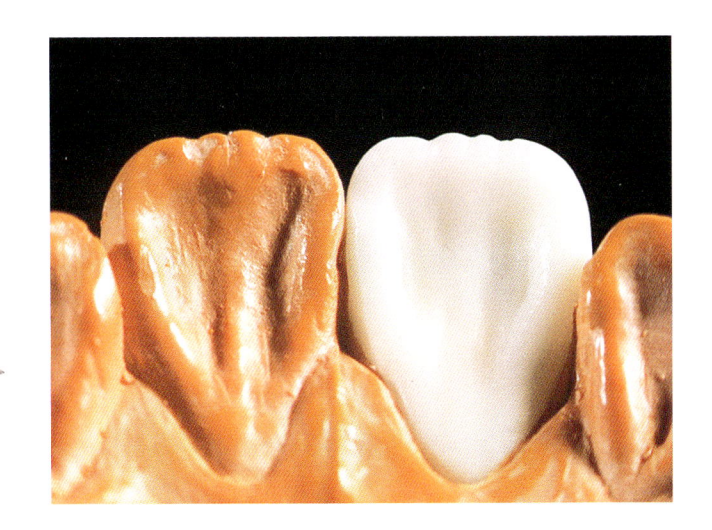

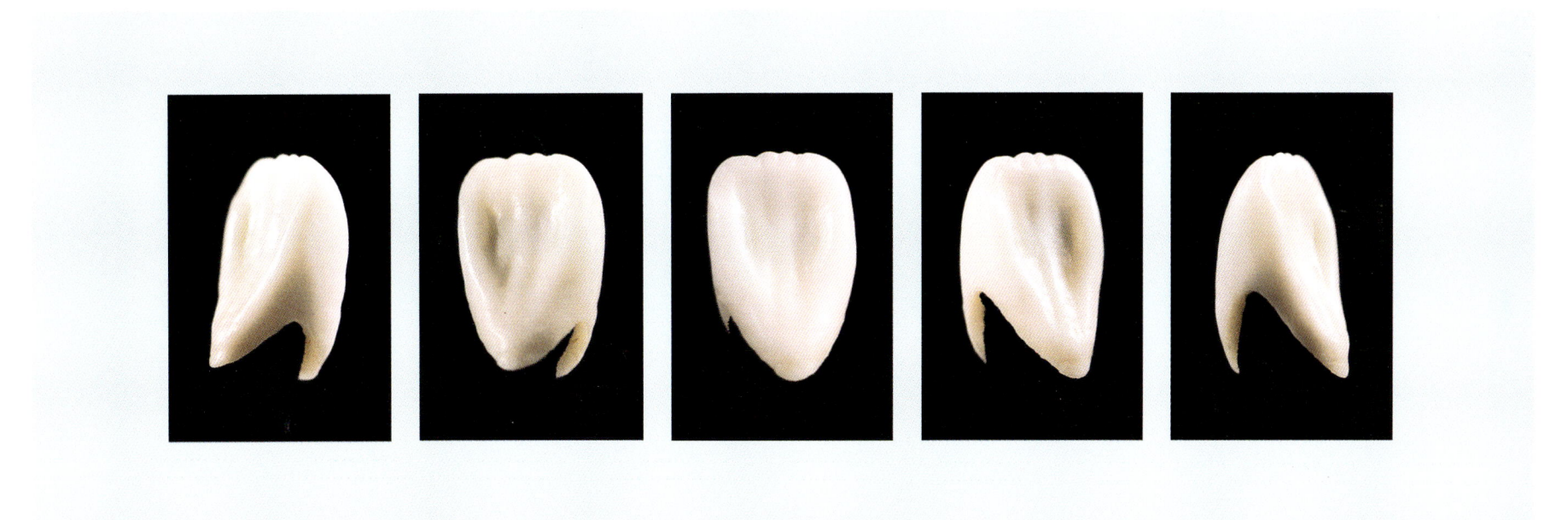

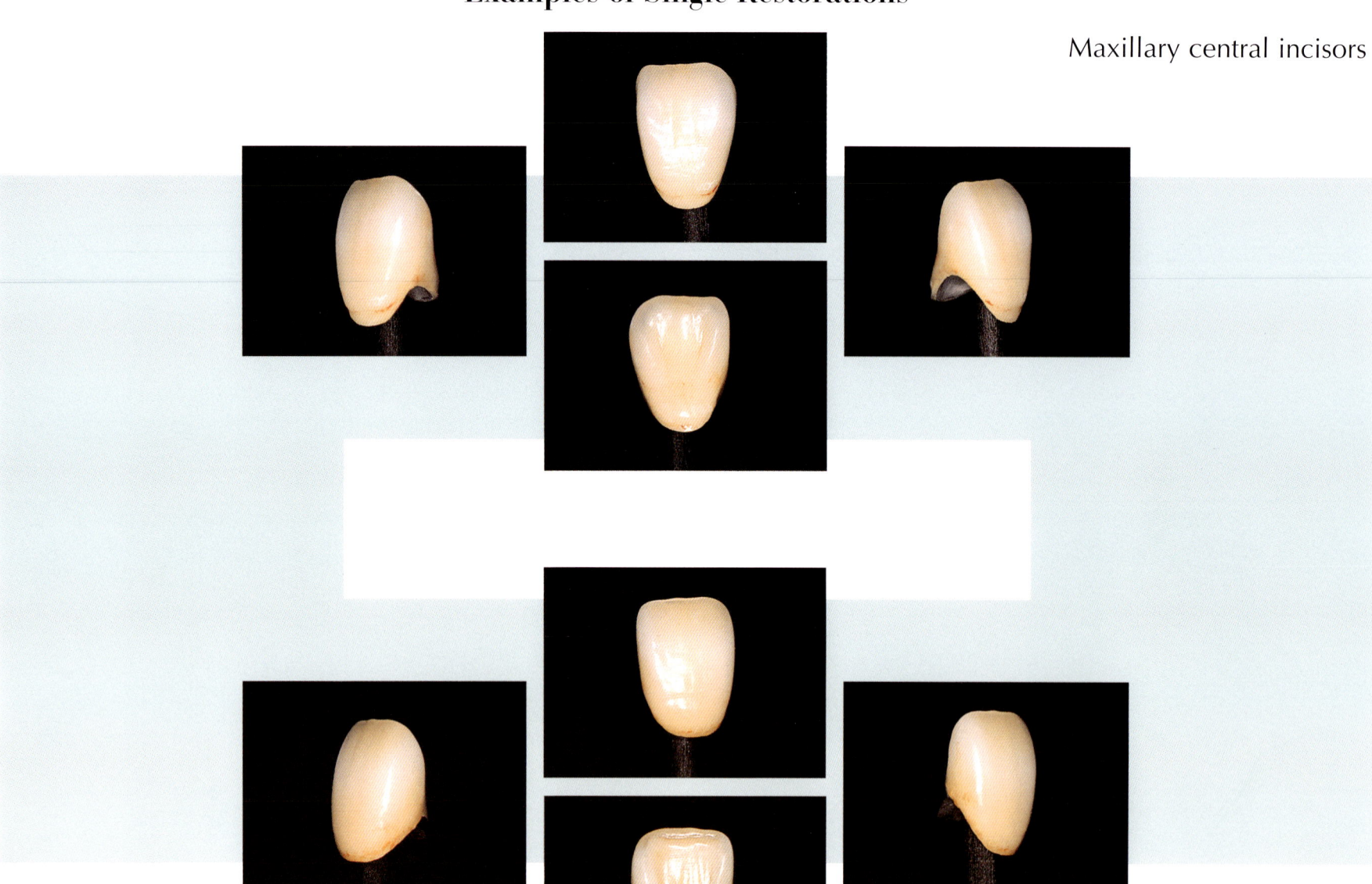

Examples of Single Restorations

Maxillary central incisors

Mandibular incisors

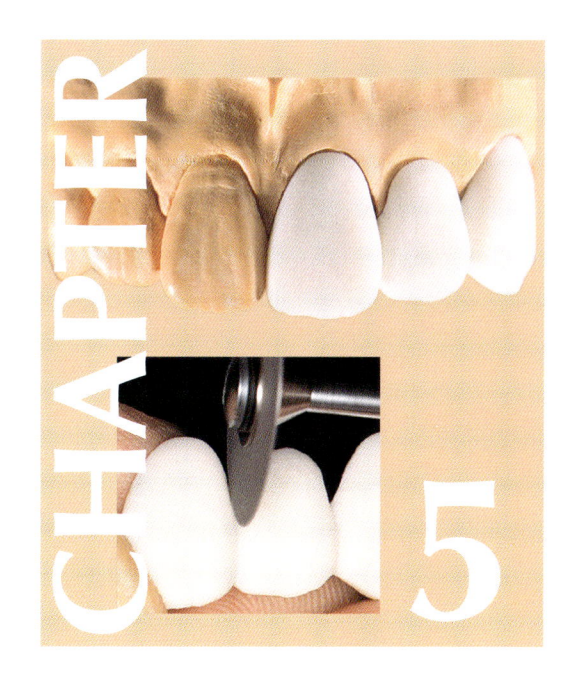

Contouring Ceramic Restorations II

Contouring a Three-Unit Fixed Partial Denture

The previous chapter presented the steps to achieve the natural morphology of a single restoration. This chapter will discuss the contouring of a fixed partial denture. In general, contouring of a fixed partial denture is similar to contouring of single restorations that adjoin each other. The result of treating the fixed partial denture as a composition of single restorations is the proper three-dimensional position of the contact points and embrasure spaces and, in the end, a natural, morphologic shape.

On the other hand, contouring of a fixed partial denture involves not only contouring of a single restoration to harmonize with the existing surrounding dentition alignment but also forming tooth alignment. Under the umbrella of tooth alignment are mesiodistal alignment balance, buccolingual relationship between lip and teeth, direction of the long axis of the roots, the length of the incisal edges, and harmony with the smile line. Therefore, a thorough knowledge of denture setup techniques is essential for mastering ceramic restorations.

A fundamental component in a fixed partial denture is the connector, which has a relatively large surface, unlike natural teeth or single restorations, which have contact points that occupy a small area. Fabricating a connector that provides the illusion of a small surface area, despite its true dimensions, is a technical challenge.

As discussed in chapter 4, good instrument selection is important for proper contouring. This chapter will also discuss instruments, including Shofu's Dura Green Stones, that are used for contouring single restorations, and diamond points, which are not required but come in shapes that promote optimal outcome.

Instruments for polishing the proximal areas of a fixed partial denture are different from those used for single restorations. The sequence of contouring (gross grinding, intermediate finishing, finishing) is the same as for single restorations and must be strictly followed because the most important factor in fabricating the proper three-dimensional shape of a fixed partial denture is a step-by-step accurate reproduction of individual tooth morphology.

ch 5 | 81

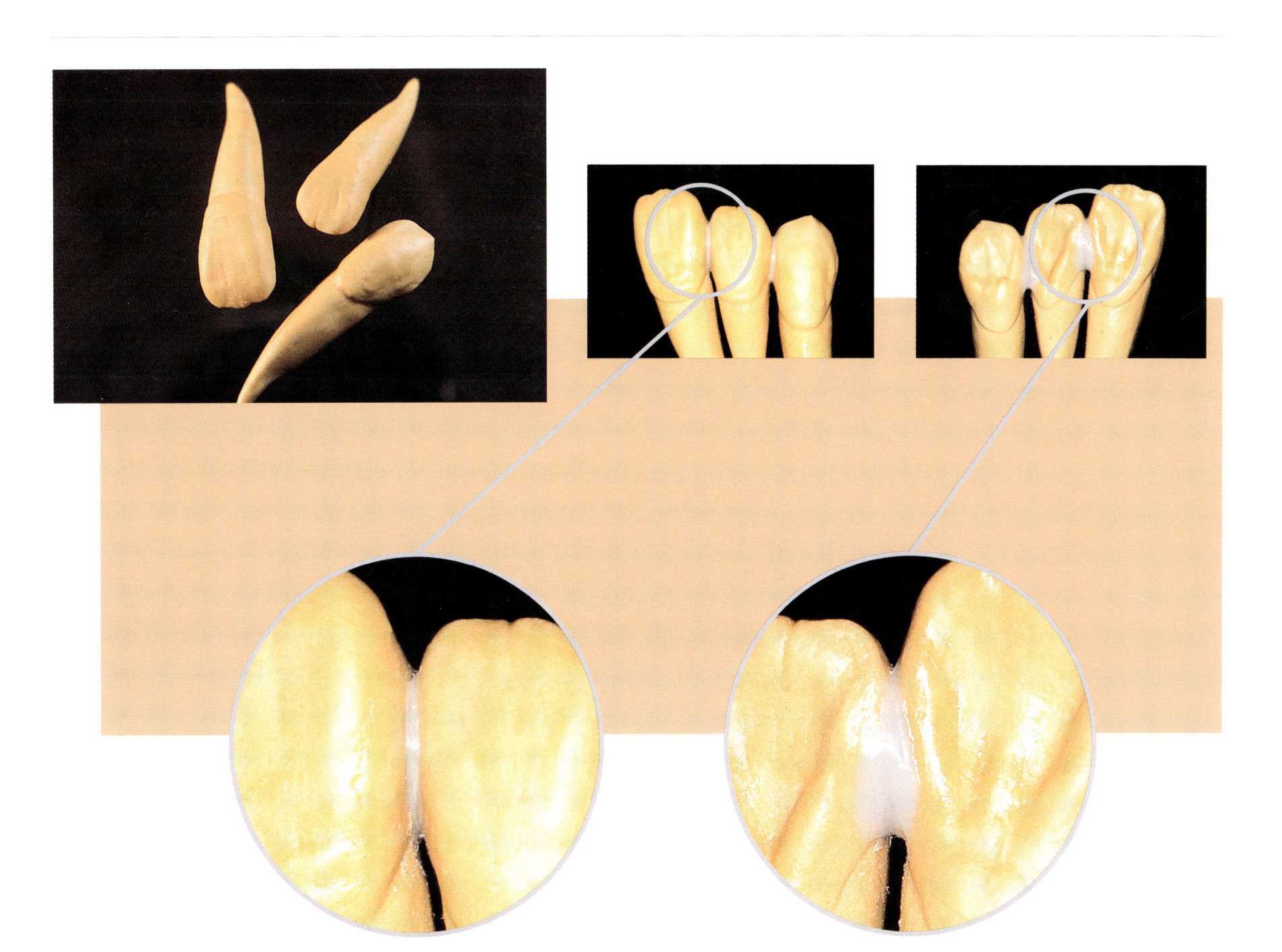

Gross Contouring I: Incisal Edge Length and Three-Plane Labial Composition

Fig 1a

Fig 1b

Fig 1c

Fig 1d

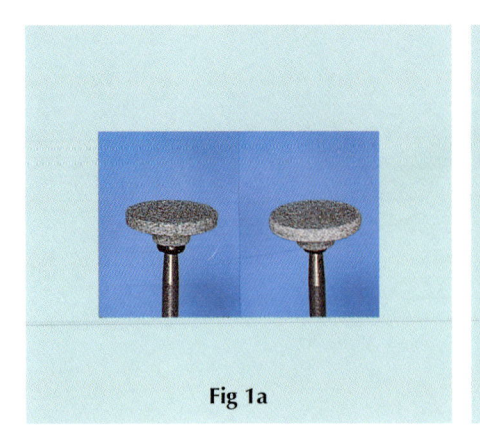

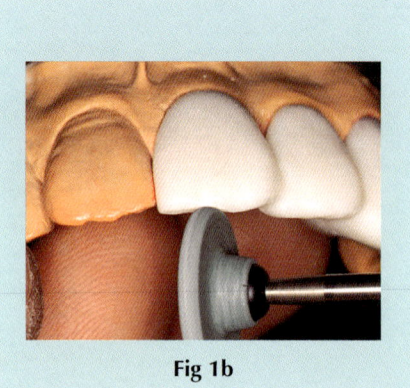

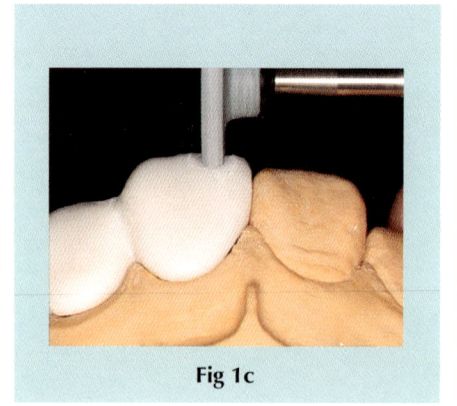

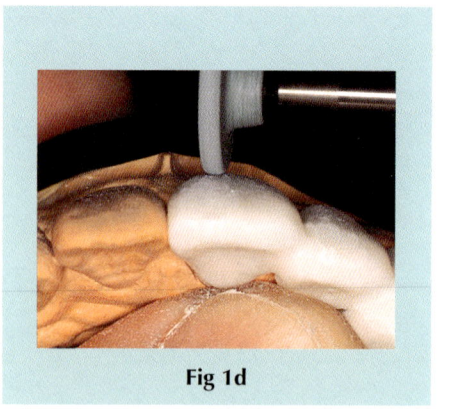

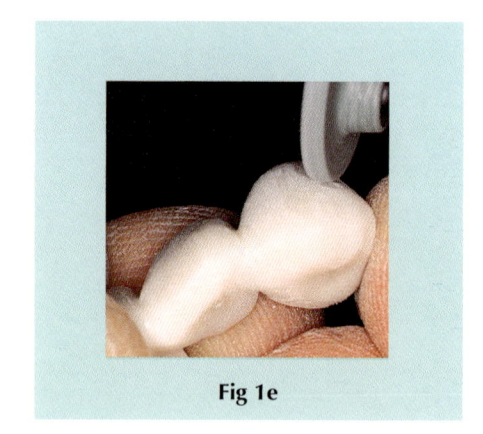

Fig 1e

Fig 1a Modify a Shofu Dura Green Stone No. WH6 *(left)* with a Shofu Abrasive Dresser by rounding off its corner *(right)*.

Fig 1b After adjusting the proximal contact point in the same manner described for a single restoration, use the smile line as a guide to adjust the incisal edge length of all teeth being restored. In this stage, angle the Dura Green Stone as shown; to contour the incisal edges, incline the instrument to the lingual. Rotate the instrument toward the lingual (not away from it) to avoid chipping the porcelain.

Fig 1c From a cervical view, adjust the contour of the incisal quarter of the buccal surfaces of the central and lateral incisors.

Fig 1d From an incisal view, adjust the contour of both the middle half and the cervical quarter of the buccal surfaces.

Fig 1e As in Fig 1d, from a distoincisal view, contour the distocervical aspect of the canine.

Fig 1f A stone cast of a typical natural tooth demonstrates the three-plane labial composition.

Fig 1g A distal view of a stone cast of a typical alignment of natural teeth demonstrates the angle of the canine distally and the three-plane labial composition of the central and lateral incisors.

Figs 1h and 1i Fixed partial denture after adjustment of incisal edge length and formation of the three-plane labial composition.

Fig 1h Labial view. With the smile line as a guide, the incisal edge length has been grossly adjusted and balanced.

Fig 1i Incisal view. The mesiodistal alignment and buccolingual contour have been grossly adjusted.

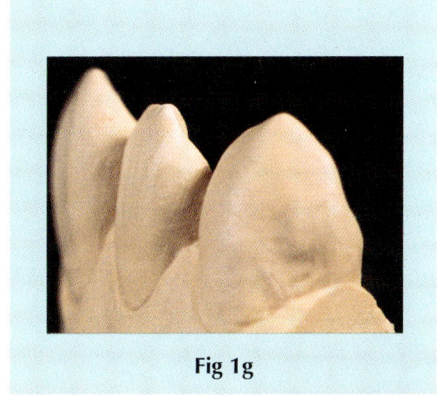

Emphasis

In this step, the shape and alignment of each tooth in the denture is grossly defined. Tooth length, mesiodistal width, and buccolingual thickness should be oversized.

The smile line should be used as a guide to establish the incisal edge length, and the contralateral teeth should be used as a reference to align the buccolingual position.

Forming the three-plane labial composition and the twist of the crown determines the buccolingual position of each of these three surfaces. The lingual inclination of the incisal quarter of the buccal surface is best contoured from a cervical view, whereas the cervical contour is best formed from an incisal view.

Although establishing individuality for each tooth is important, balancing the smile line is even more critical. Therefore, using the smile line as a guide to adjust the incisal edge length is of utmost importance.

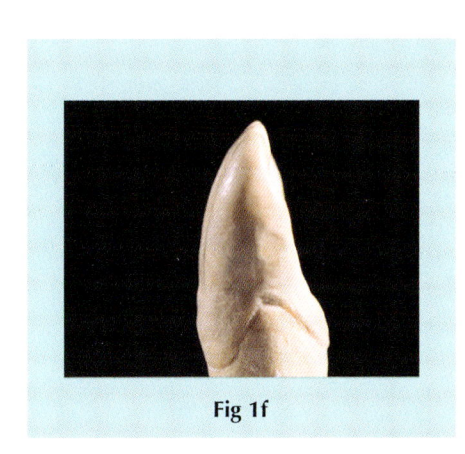

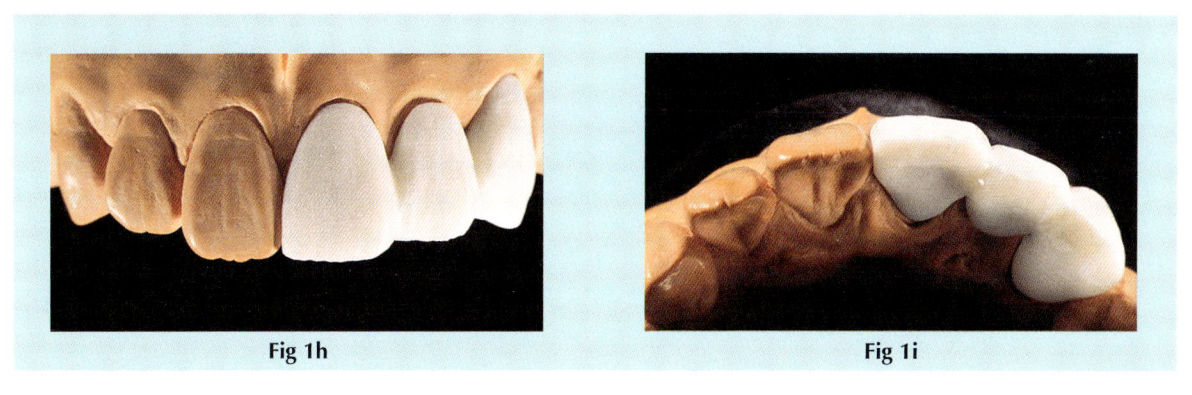

Gross Contouring II: Midline Area (Interproximal Space)

Fig 2a

Fig 2b — Interproximal space / Contact point

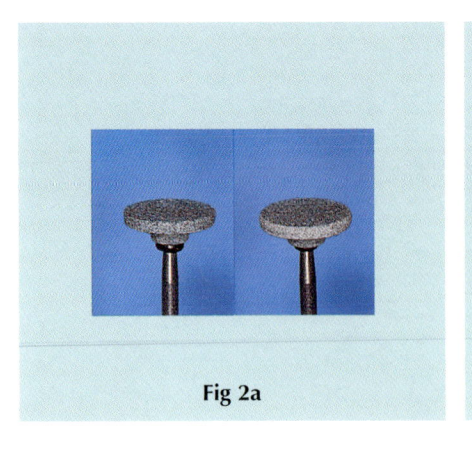

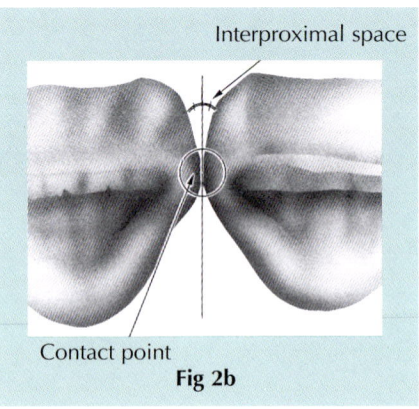

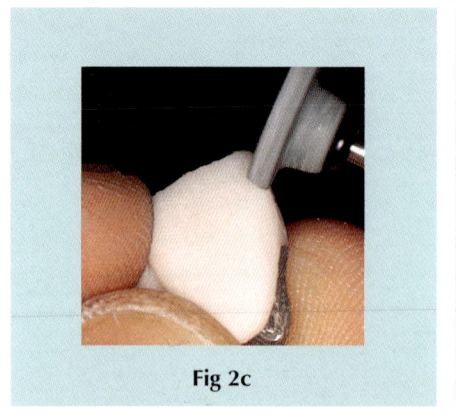

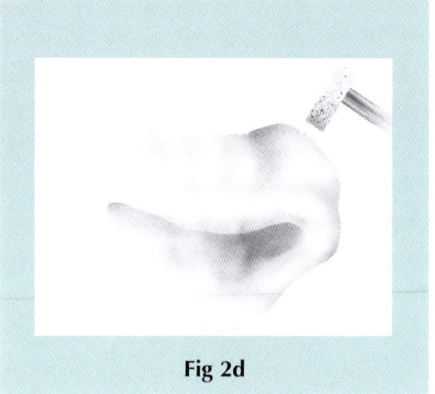

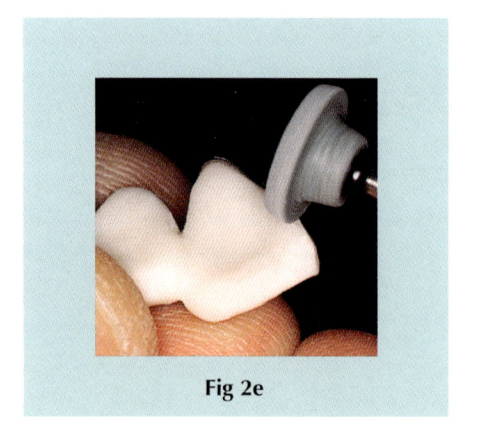

Fig 2c

Fig 2d

Fig 2e

Fig 2a Modify a Shofu Dura Green Stone No. WH6 *(left)* with a Shofu Abrasive Dresser by rounding off its corner *(right)*.

Fig 2b The proximal contact point of a central incisor is the contact point between the mesial walls of adjacent central incisors in the sagittal plane.

Figs 2c and 2d First determine the location of the proximal contact point of the fixed partial denture, and only then adjust the mesiolabial proximal transitional surface, also called the *interproximal opening*, to achieve symmetry between the central incisors.

Fig 2e Use the same principle to adjust the interproximal opening to form symmetry from the lingual aspect. The determined contact point is the reference point from which contouring toward the lingual takes place.

Emphasis

At this step, the location and direction of the peak of the mesial marginal ridge are used as guides to contour the proximal transitional surface of the central incisor (Fig 2g) and to accurately contour the interproximal space (Fig 2i). This contouring step is very important because this will be the reference to determine the width of the tooth and the direction of the long axis of the tooth.

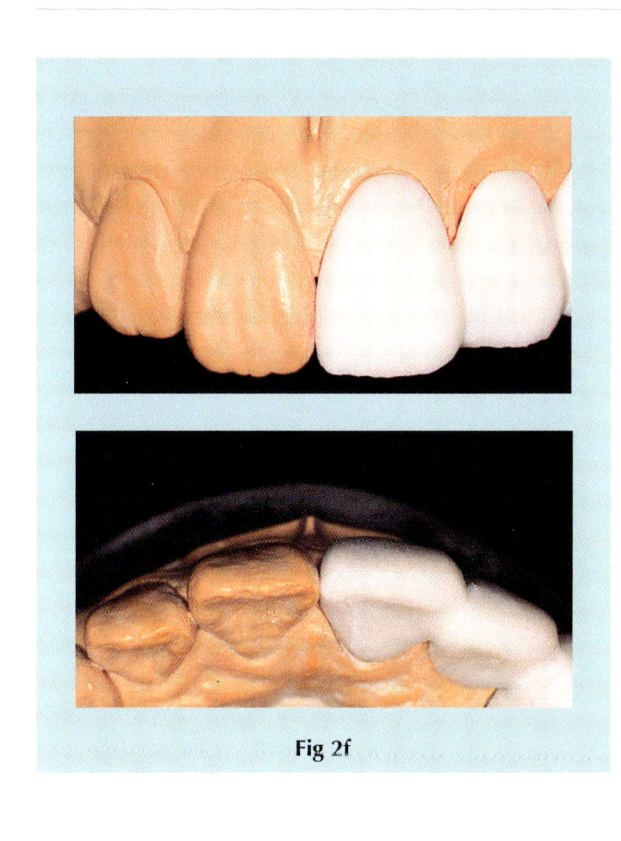

Fig 2f Fixed partial denture after adjustment of interproximal spaces. Labial view *(top)*; incisal view *(bottom)*.

Figs 2g to 2i Interrelationship between the peak of the marginal ridge, the proximal transitional surface, and the interproximal space.

Fig 2g Relationship between the peak of the mesial marginal ridge of a central incisor and the proximal transitional surface (incisal view).

Fig 2h Relationship between the direction of the peak of the mesial marginal ridge of a central incisor and the proximal transitional surface (labial view, stone cast).

Fig 2i Interproximal space (incisal view, stone cast).

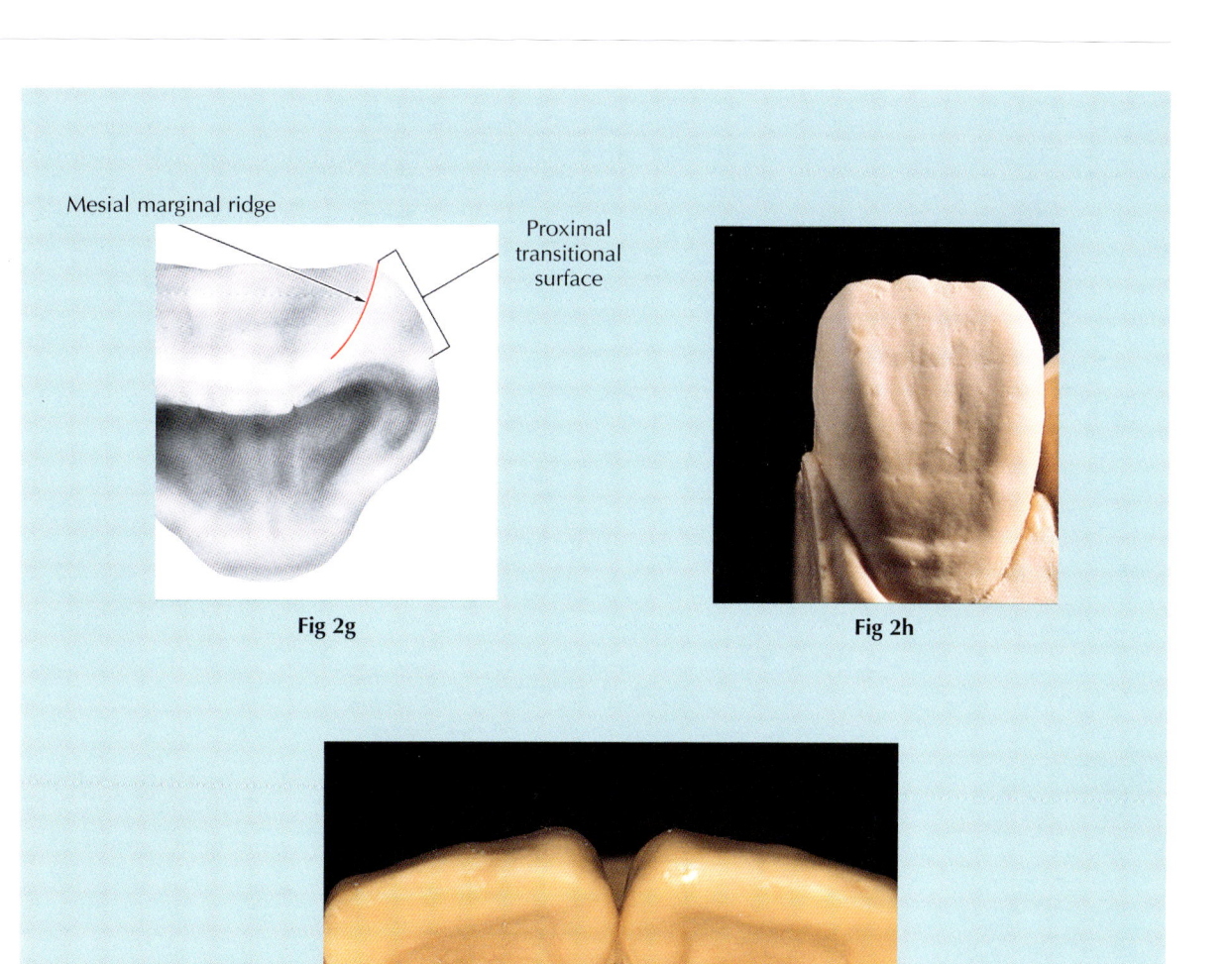

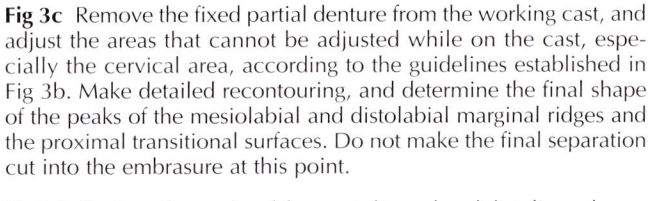

Gross Contouring III: Proximal Transitional Surfaces and Individualization

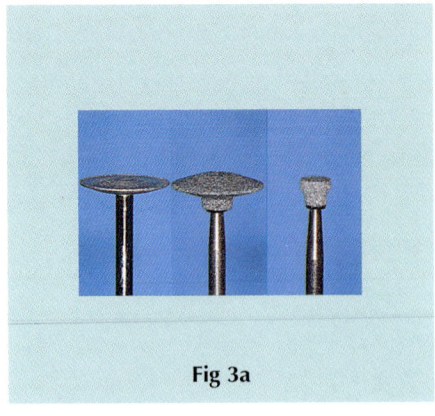

Fig 3a Diamond disk *(left)*, Shofu Dura Green Stone No. KN7 *(middle)*, and modified Shofu Dura Green Stone No. KN7 *(right)*.

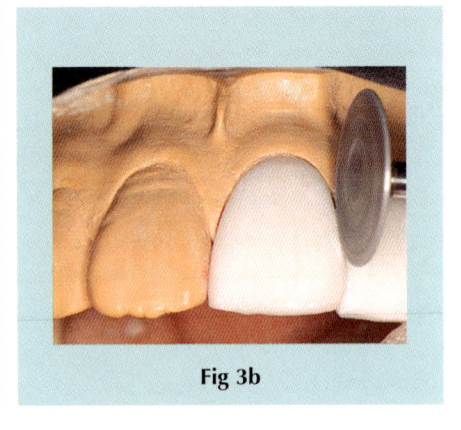

Fig 3b With the fixed partial denture seated on the cast that serves as a reference guide, adjust the peak of the mesial and distal marginal ridges and the proximal transitional surfaces. Evaluate the contour from an incisal view, comparing it to the contralateral tooth. Further adjustments to the contour, width, and long axis of each tooth can be done with the fixed partial denture off the working cast.

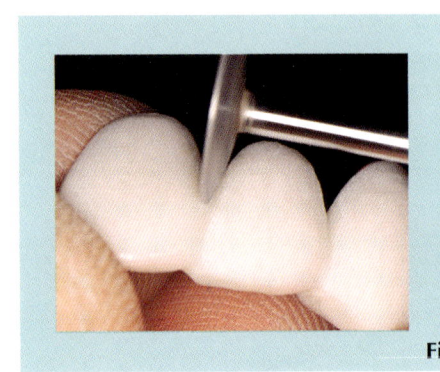

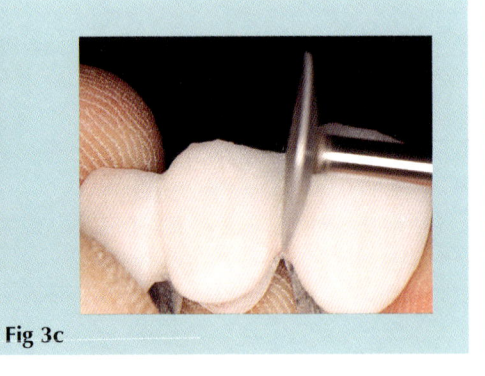

Fig 3a

Fig 3b

Fig 3c

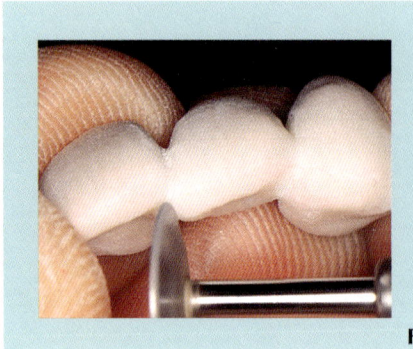

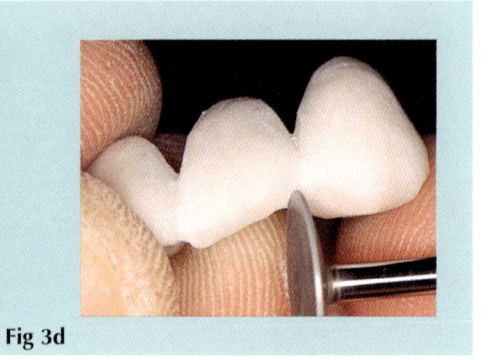

Fig 3d

Fig 3c Remove the fixed partial denture from the working cast, and adjust the areas that cannot be adjusted while on the cast, especially the cervical area, according to the guidelines established in Fig 3b. Make detailed recontouring, and determine the final shape of the peaks of the mesiolabial and distolabial marginal ridges and the proximal transitional surfaces. Do not make the final separation cut into the embrasure at this point.

Fig 3d Contour the peaks of the mesiolingual and distolingual marginal ridges. Establish the proximal transitional surface of each tooth in the same manner as in Fig 3c.

Fig 3e Further modify the Shofu Dura Green Stone No. KN7 (Fig 3a, *right*) with a Shofu Abrasive Dresser, and grossly contour the lingual fossa pass through the proximal surface.

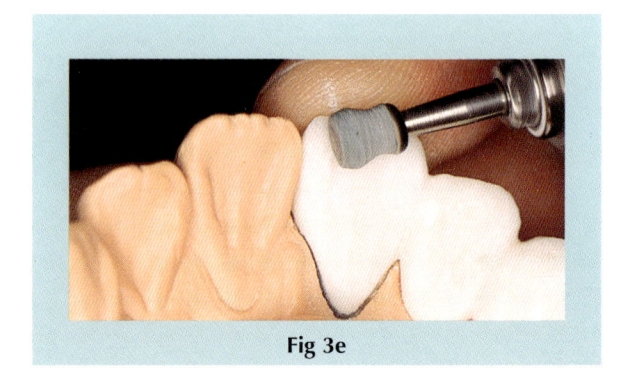

Fig 3e

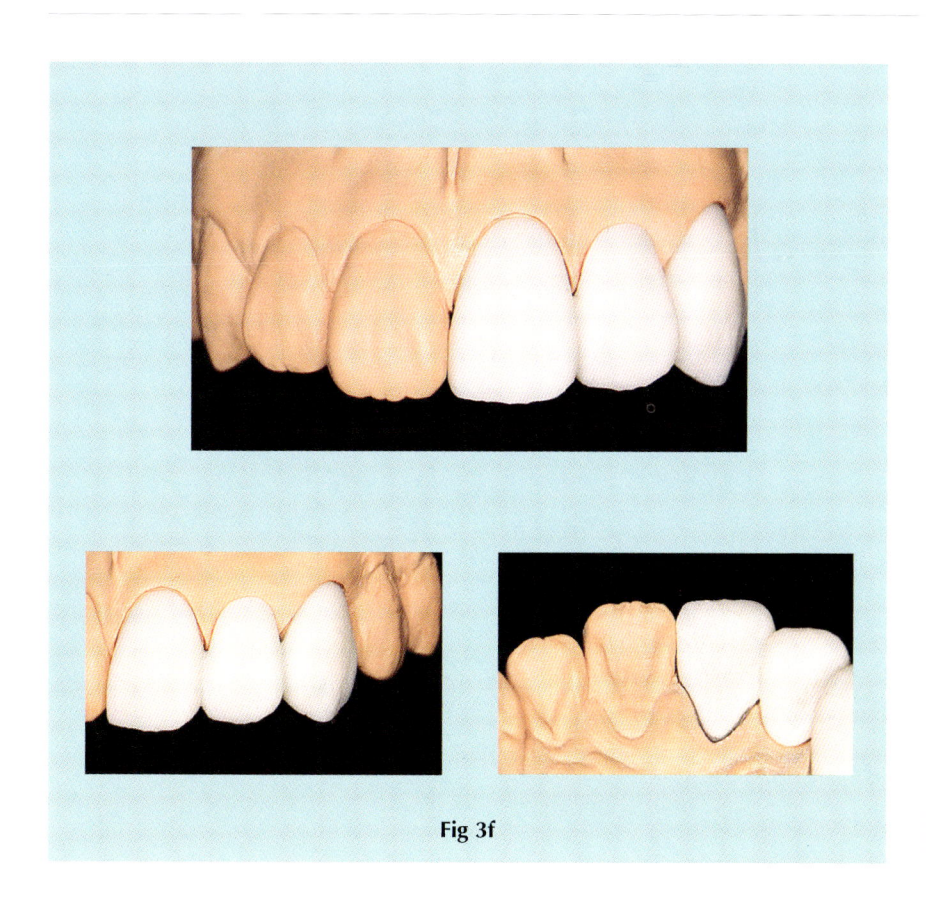

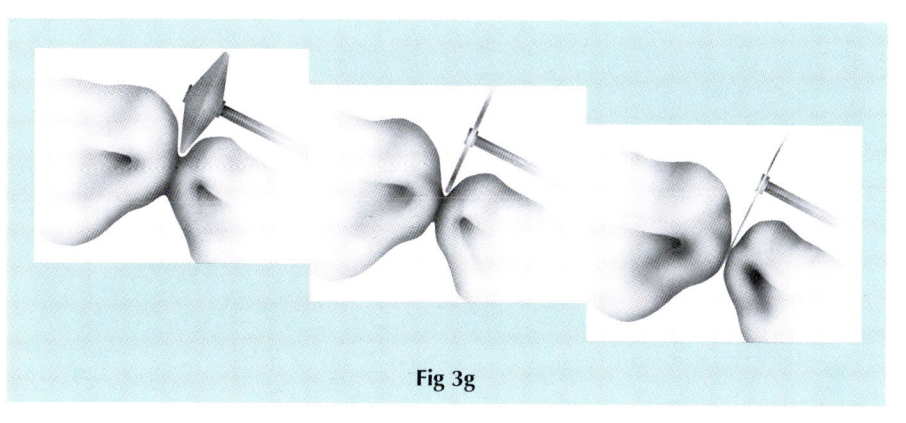

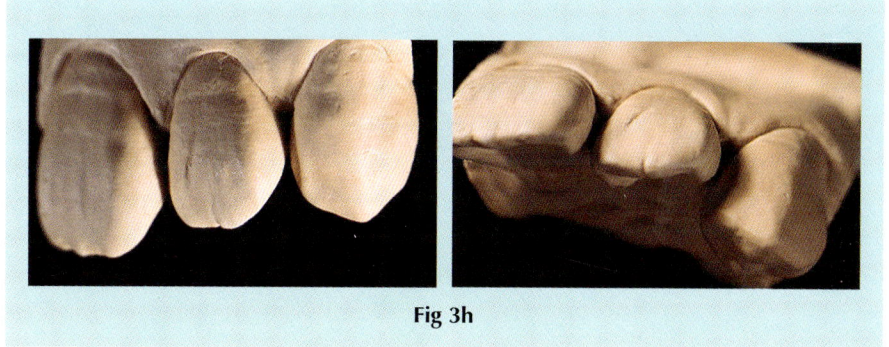

Fig 3f The fixed partial denture after contouring of the proximal transitional surfaces and individualization. Labial view *(top)*; labial-lateral view *(left)*; lingual view *(right)*.

Fig 3g Schematic illustrations of the steps for contouring a proximal area and the different shapes of the instruments used. Shofu Dura Green Stone No. KN7 *(left)*; Shofu Sintadisc S61T (0.3-mm thickness) *(middle)*; Shofu Sintadisc S61UT (0.15-mm thickness) *(right)*.

Fig 3h A stone cast of natural dentition showing the form of the interproximal area. Labial-lateral view *(left)*; incisal view *(right)*.

Emphasis

The contouring of each mesial and distal marginal ridge determines the width of each tooth that the fixed partial denture restores. The ridge in turn determines the location and direction of each peak, and the contralateral tooth serves as a guide. Individualization and separation, along with contouring of the proximal transitional surfaces, are used to determine the width of each tooth in the denture.

Use of different point shapes (Fig 3g) helps to achieve the shape of natural dentition shown in Fig 3h.

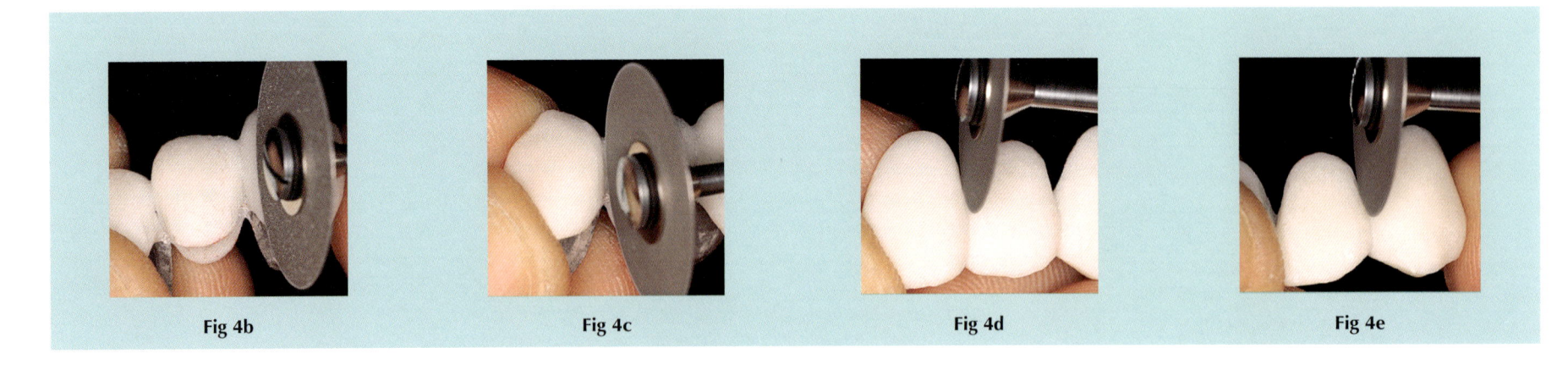

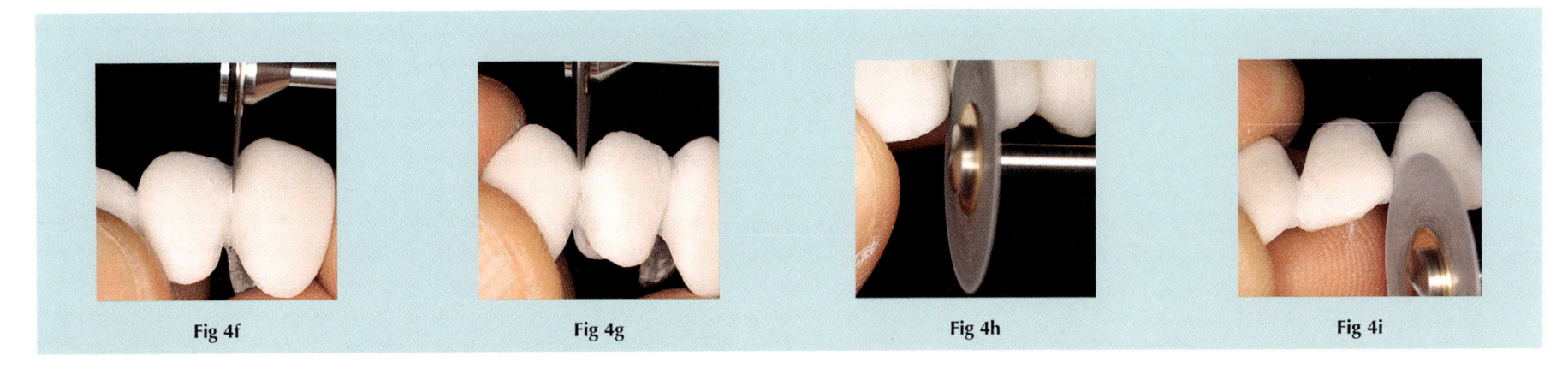

Intermediate Finishing I: Proximal Transitional Surface

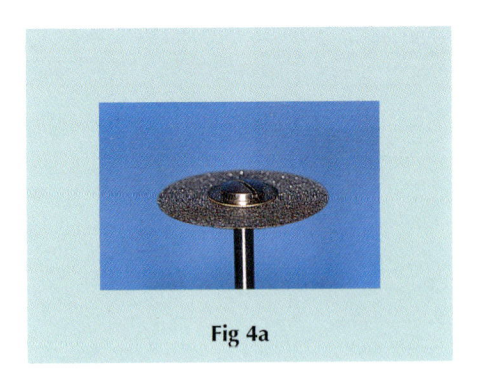

Fig 4a Shofu Sintadisc S61T (0.3-mm thickness).

Figs 4b to 4e Use the Shofu Sintadisc to contour the proximal transitional surface from the connector to the cervical area.

Figs 4b and 4c To contour distal proximal transitional surfaces of the central and lateral incisors, hold the prosthesis in a cervical view.

Figs 4d and 4e To contour the mesial proximal transitional surfaces of the lateral incisor and canine, hold the prosthesis in an incisal view.

Figs 4f to 4i Use the Shofu Sintadisc to contour the proximal transitional area from the connector to the incisal edge and the lingual side.

Figs 4f and 4g Hold the denture in a cervical view to contour the incisal side of the distal proximal transitional surface of the central and lateral incisors and to form the incisal interproximal space.

Figs 4h and 4i Hold the denture in an incisal view to contour the lingual aspect of the incisal interproximal space.

Fig 4a

Fig 4b

Fig 4c

Fig 4d

Fig 4e

Fig 4f

Fig 4g

Fig 4h

Fig 4i

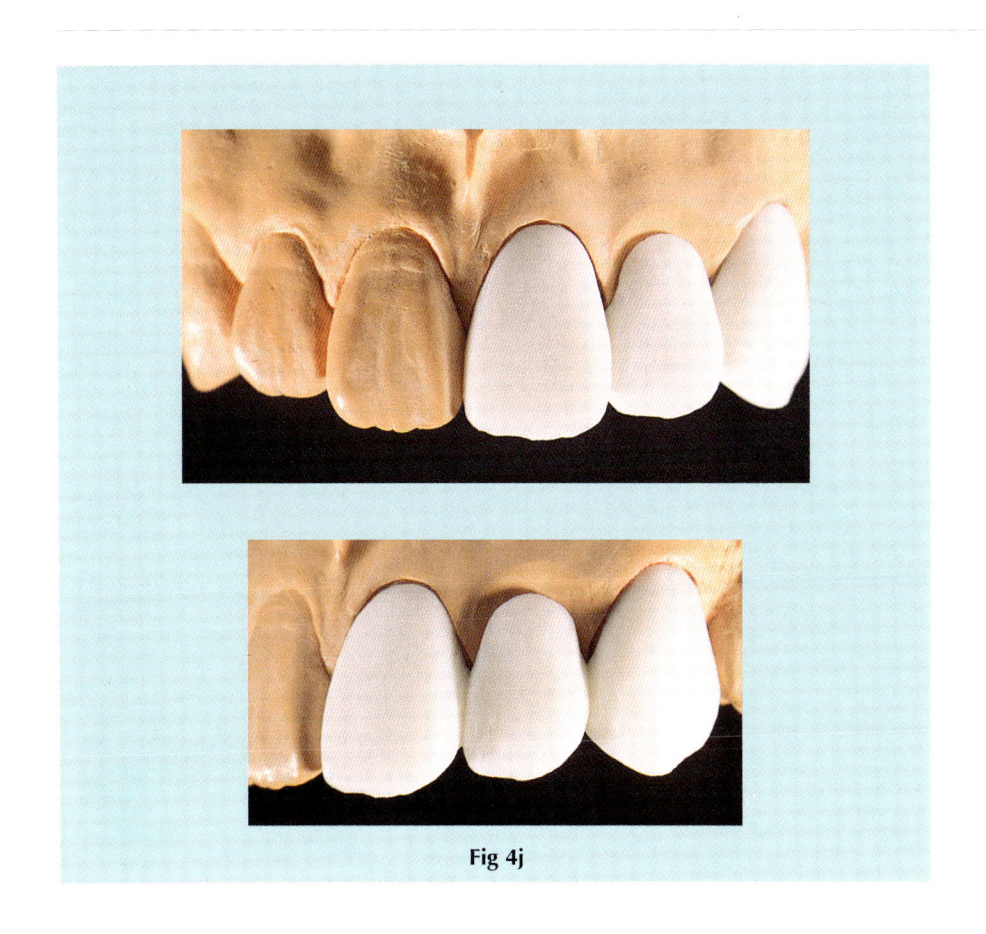

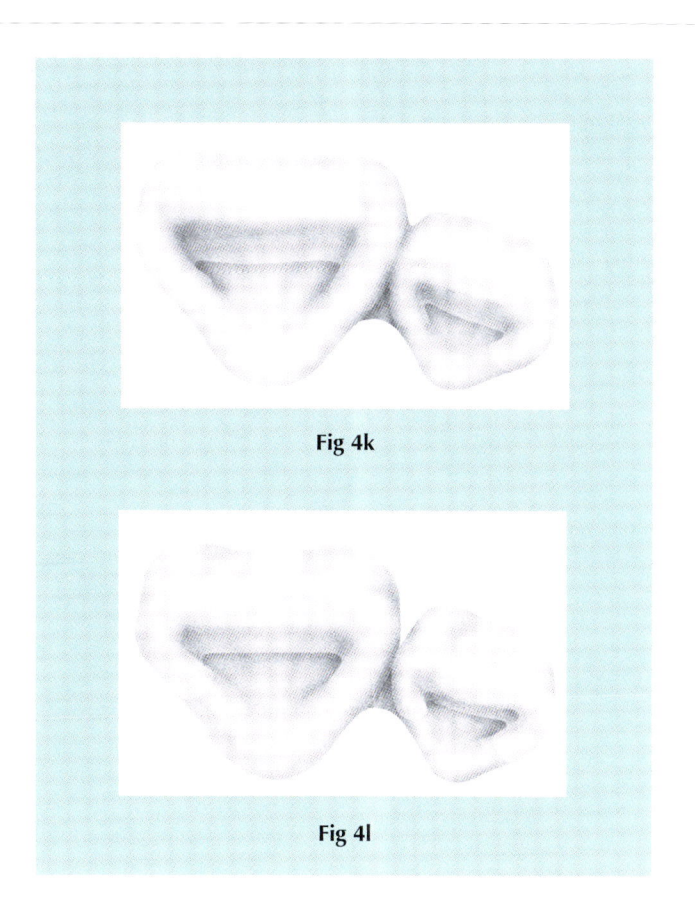

Fig 4j The fixed partial denture after contouring of each proximal transitional surface with the Shofu Sintadisc. Labial view *(top)*; labial-lateral view *(bottom)*.

Figs 4k and 4l Schematic illustrations of the contouring of the proximal transitional surface.

Fig 4k Preliminary contouring of the proximal area with the Shofu Sintadisc.

Fig 4l Final contouring of the proximal area.

Emphasis

The final separation cut into the embrasure (Fig 4l) is not completed at this step; thus, instead, the disk is used to contour the proximal transitional surfaces as well as to deepen the proximal area. Therefore, use of the front and back surfaces of the disk, rather than the cutting edge, is recommended. A thinner disk will be used later to achieve the depth shown in Fig 4l. At this stage, the level of separation shown in Fig 4k should be achieved. The contouring of the proximal transitional surfaces and the interproximal spaces should not be completed.

Intermediate Finishing II: Labial Ridges

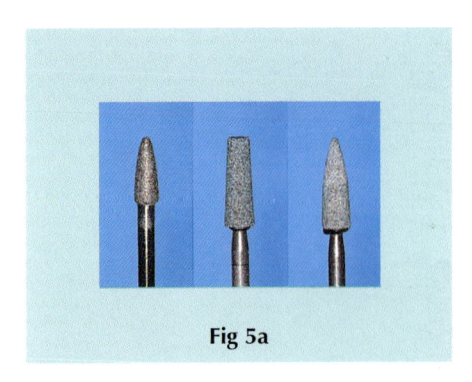

Fig 5a Use a tapered diamond bur *(left)* or modify a Shofu Dura Green Stone No. TC4 *(middle)* to a bullet shape *(right)*.

Fig 5b For final contouring of the incisal quarter, hold the fixed partial denture in an cervical view.

Fig 5c From the midlabial to the cervical, complete the final contouring of the twist of the tooth crown and the height of each ridge. Establish the proper relationship between the restoration and the gingival tissues. Also contour the transverse ridges of the cervical area.

Fig 5d Remove the denture from the working cast, and finish the final contour of the cervical area close to the margins and the margin area.

Fig 5e Contour the area of the labial grooves, defining the location and the depth of the grooves accurately. The grooves will serve as the guide for forming the labial ridges.

Fig 5f Contour the internal slope from the groove to the peak of the ridge, and determine the form and direction of the marginal ridges. Note the position of the instrument used for finishing the mesiolabial marginal ridge of the central incisor *(left)* and the lateral incisor *(right)*.

Fig 5g Complete the contouring of the proximal transitional surfaces of the marginal ridges. Note the position of the instrument used for finishing the distolabial marginal ridge of the central incisor *(left)* and the lateral incisor *(right)*.

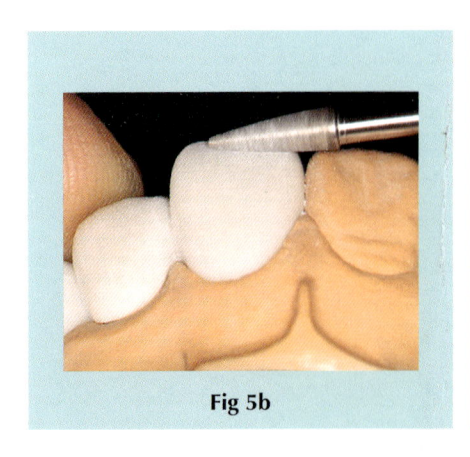

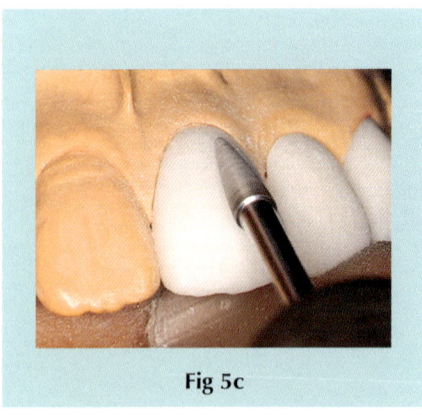

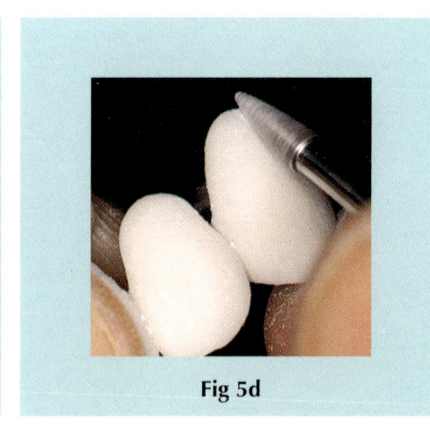

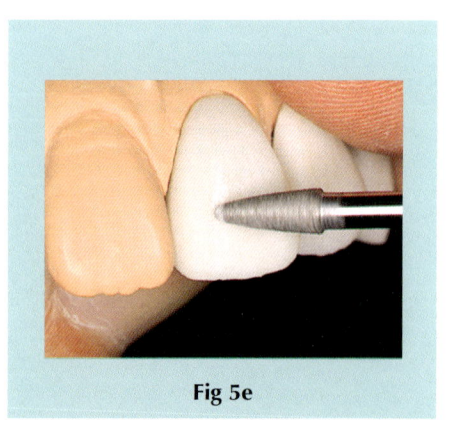

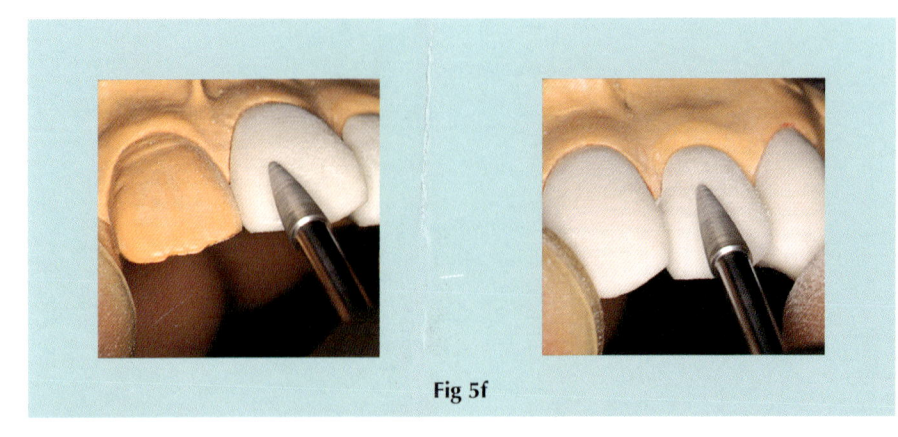

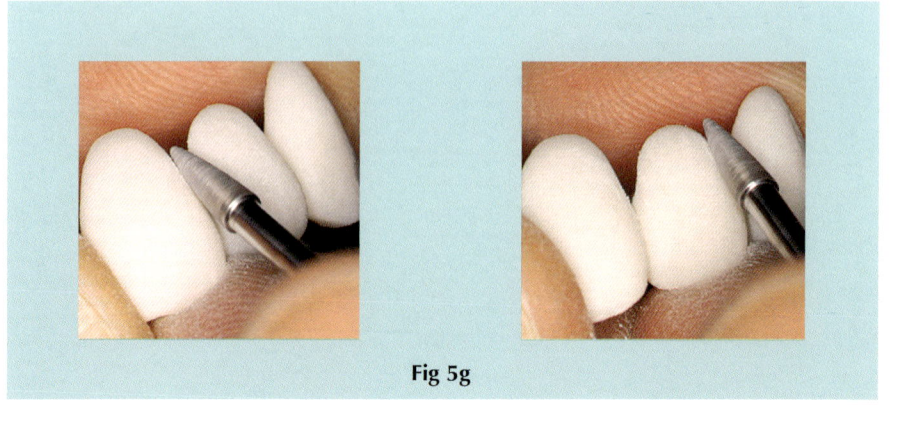

Fig 5a

Fig 5b

Fig 5c

Fig 5d

Fig 5e

Fig 5f

Fig 5g

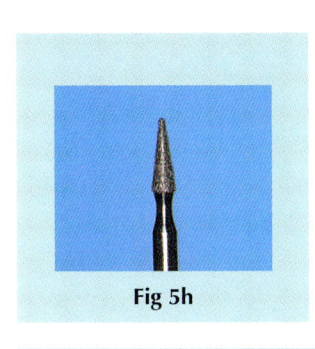

Fig 5h Use the Brasseler needle No. 852-023 (diamond point).

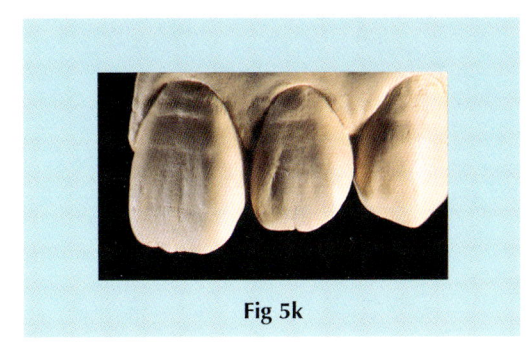

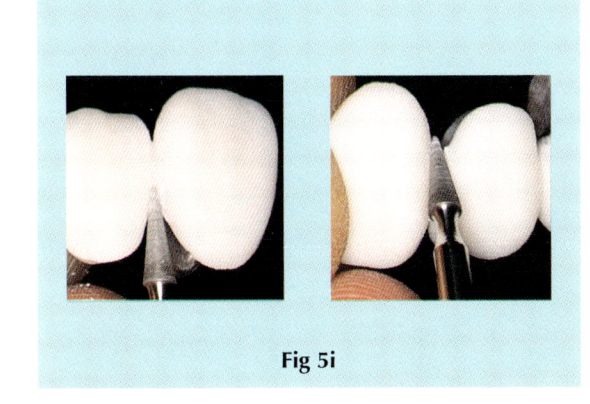

Fig 5i Contour the deeper area of the proximal transitional surface and the cervical area of the proximal transitional surface to complete the finishing of the marginal ridge.

Fig 5j Contour in detail the incisal aspect of the proximal transitional surface of the marginal ridge, and finish the incisal line angles.

Fig 5k A stone cast of natural dentition demonstrates continuity in form from the labial groove to the inner slope of the marginal ridge, to the peak of the ridge, to the proximal transitional surface, and to the proximal contact point.

Fig 5l Fixed partial denture after contouring of each ridge and the incisal line angles using Brasseler needle No. 852-023. Labial view *(top)*; labial-lateral view *(bottom)*.

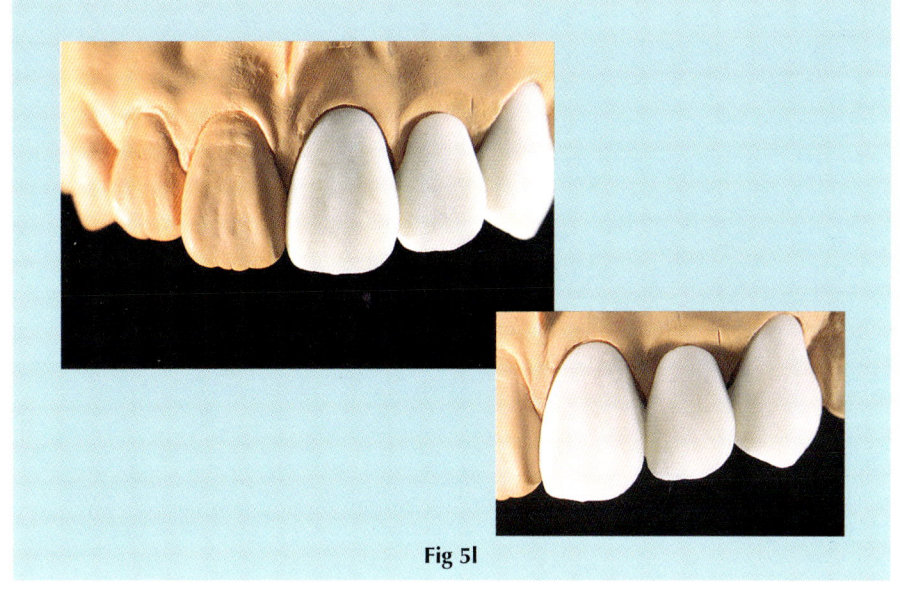

Emphasis

After the width and the proximal transitional surface of each tooth have been roughly determined, detailed contouring of the proximal transitional surface is started, using a diamond point. At this step, the final shape and surface characteristics, such as the direction of the labial ridge, the contour of the cervical area, the twist of the tooth crown, etc, are formed.

It is important to contour the marginal ridges from both the mid-labial surface and the proximal transitional surface. The subtle surfaces are formed toward the peaks of the ridges to obtain the three-dimensional shape. This technique should also be used for other ridges, including the central ridge. To form the ridge, adjustments should be made from both sides of the ridge toward the peak. Grooves and pits are created by accumulation and continuity of each ridge. As a result, individuality and three-dimensional form are achieved.

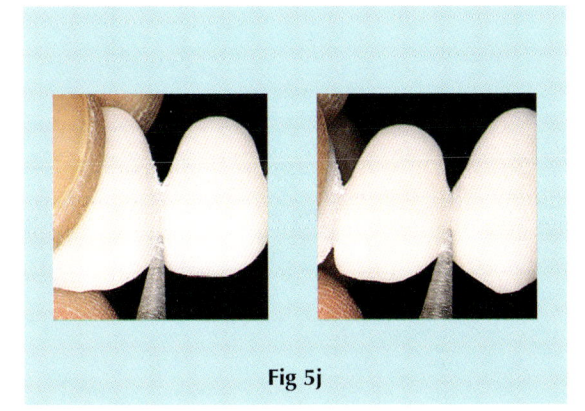

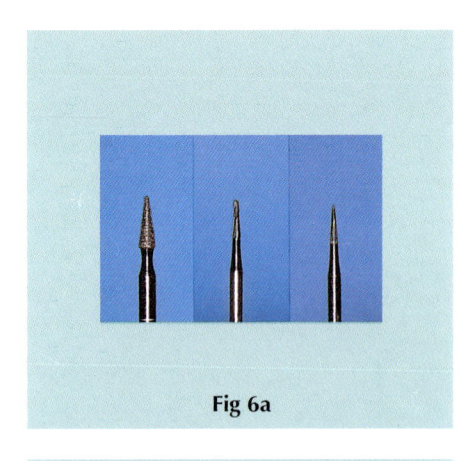

Finishing I: Proximal Area and Lingual Grooves

Fig 6a Brasseler needle No. 852-023 *(left)*; Shofu Robot Carbide Finisher FG *(middle)*; modified nonedge carbide bur *(right)*.

Fig 6b Smooth the deepest cervical area of the connector with a nonedge bur, and form the cervical line at the interproximal area.

Fig 6c Form the deepest incisal area of the proximal area from the labial and the lingual sides with a nonedge bur. Also form the proximal groove in this area.

Fig 6d Form the deepest area of the lingual groove with a nonedge bur. With the Brasseler needle No. 852-023, smooth the sharp corner that the nonedge bur created.

Fig 6e Use the Brasseler needle No. 852-023 to form the lingual fossa, which escapes to the area of the proximal line angle of the incisal edge through the lingual marginal ridge.

Fig 6f The cervical line and the subtle morphology of the proximal surface emerges from the cervical line.

Figs 6g and 6h Contouring mainly from an incisal direction, use a Shofu Sintadisc S61UT to finalize the deepest area of the incisal aspect of the interproximal proximal surface.

Fig 6g Shofu Sintadisc S61UT (0.15-mm thickness).

Fig 6h Illustration.

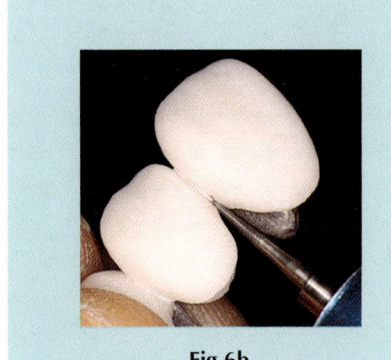

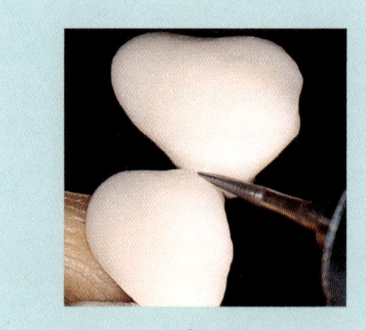

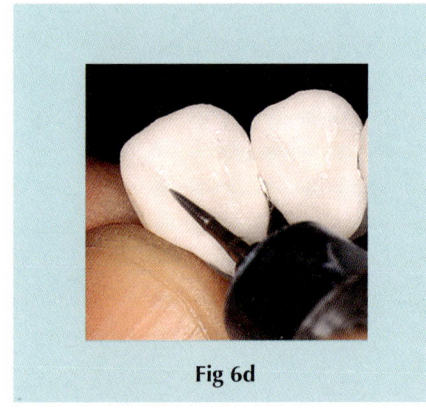

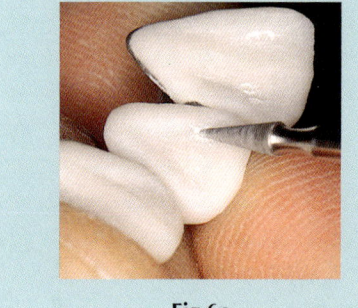

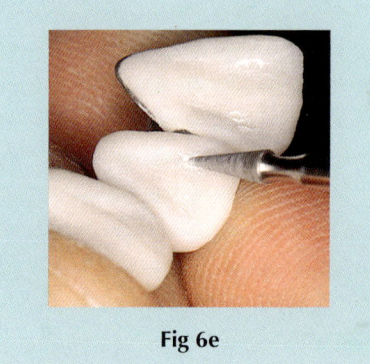

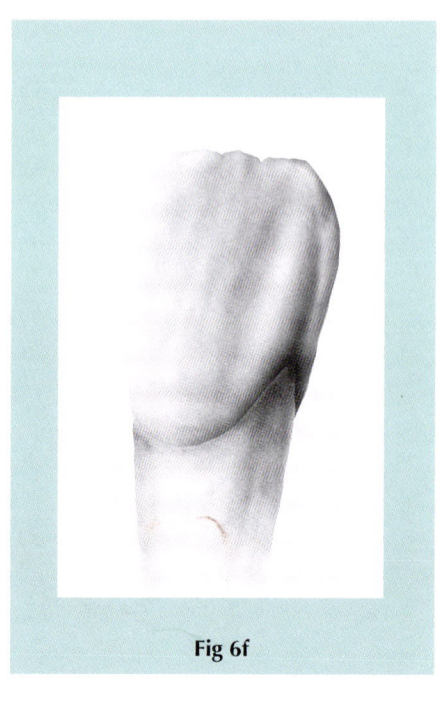

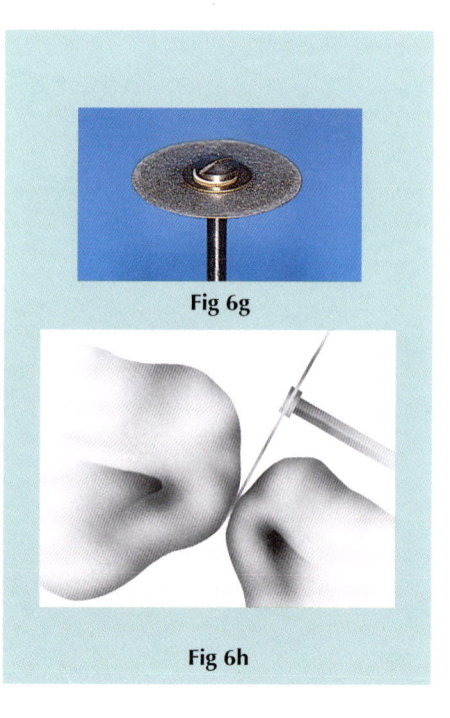

Fig 6i

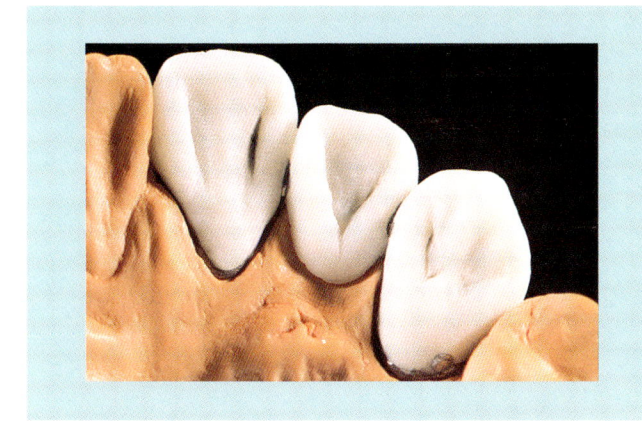

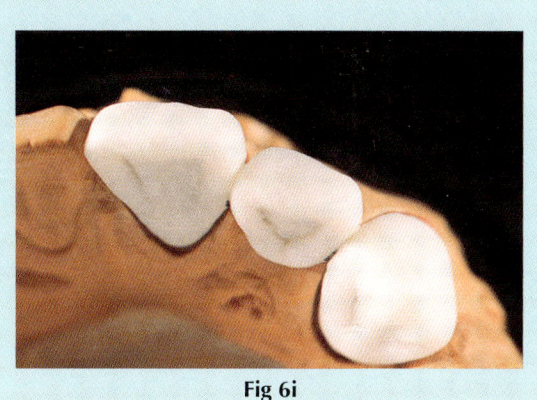

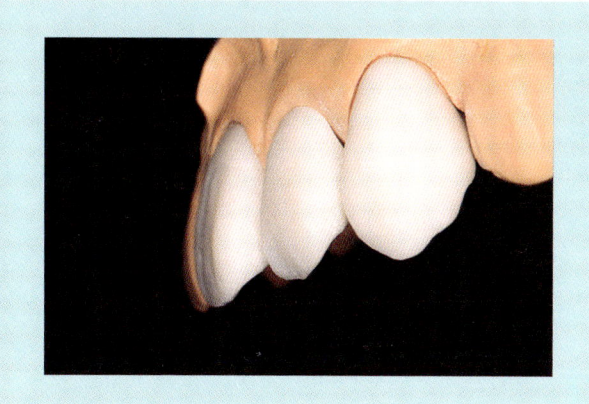

Emphasis

The morphology of the lingual fossa determines the morphology of the incisal line angles. The lingual fossa creates an escape route to the proximal surface through the mesial and distal marginal ridges and through the peak of the lingual marginal ridge, continuing to the incisal ridge. The morphology of the incisal edge cannot be reproduced by working only on the labial side.

The lingual view of the central and lateral incisors in Fig 6j shows that the mesial and distal marginal ridges are connected to the incisal ridge and thus form part of the incisal line angle. The lateral view in Fig 6j demonstrates the role of the lingual marginal ridges in the three-dimensional form of these teeth.

Fig 6i Fixed partial denture prior to surface characterization. Lingual view *(left)*; incisal view *(middle)*; lateral view *(right)*.

Fig 6j Stone cast of natural dentition demonstrating the incisal line angle that the morphology of the lingual fossa forms extending into the incisal area. The continuation of the peak of the lingual marginal ridge to the incisal ridge is visible. Lingual view *(left)*; incisal view *(middle)*; lateral view *(right)*.

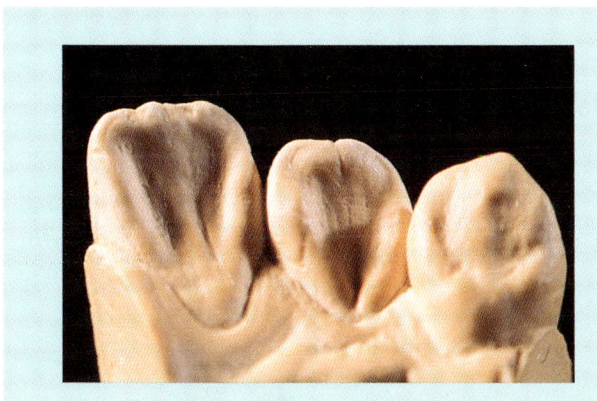

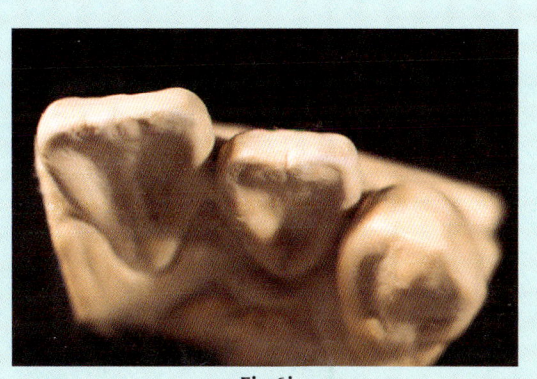

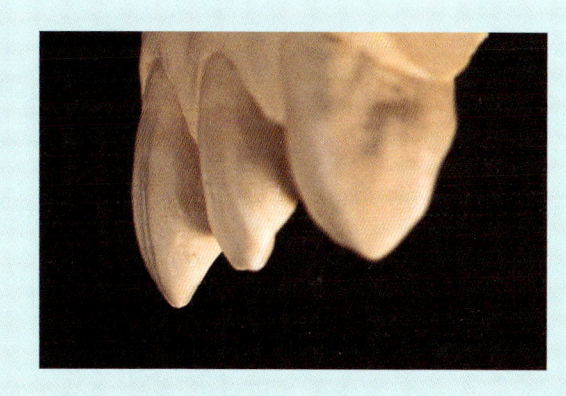

Fig 6j

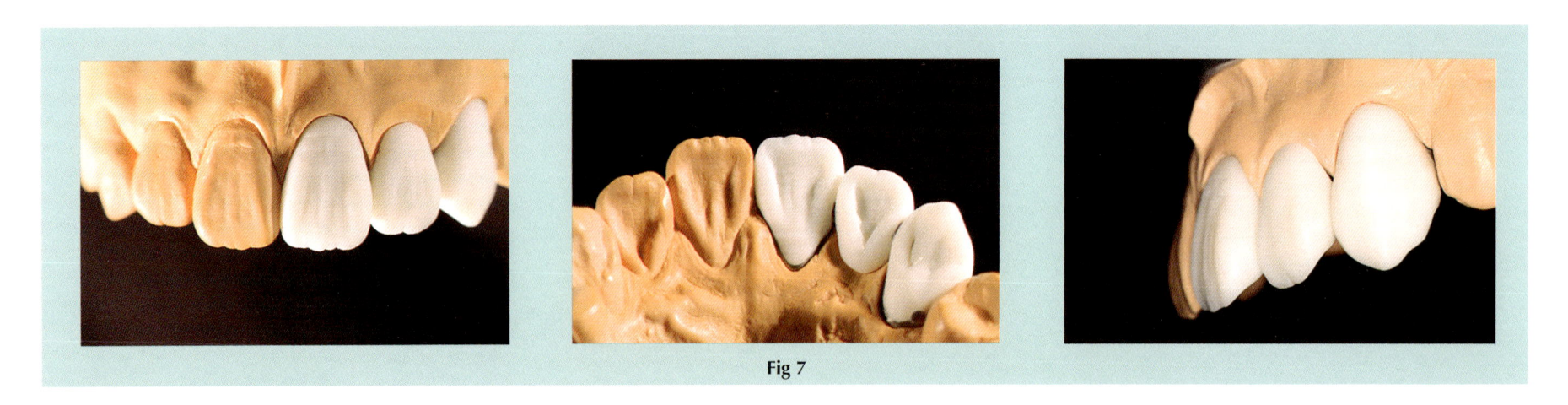

Finishing II: Surface Characterization and Polishing

Characterization

Fig 7 Fixed partial denture after contouring and surface characterization. The characterization method is the same as that used for a single restoration. Labial view *(left)*; lingual view *(middle)*; lateral view *(right)*.

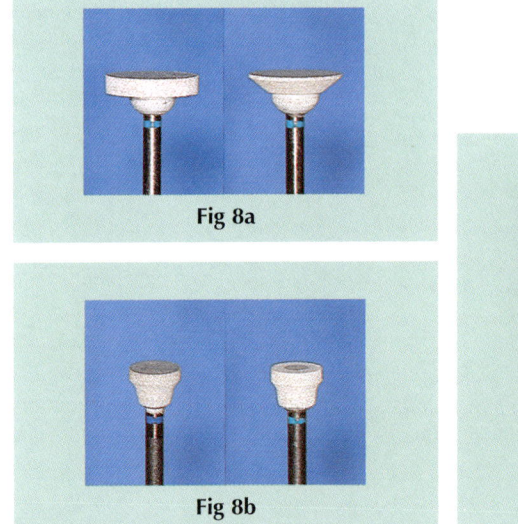

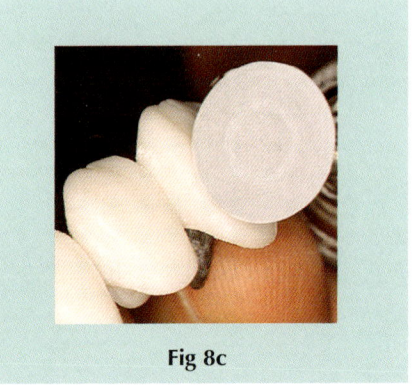

Surface polishing

Fig 8a Modify a Shofu Ceramiste Soft No. PA *(left)* with a Shofu Abrasive Dresser as shown *(right)*.

Fig 8b Modified Shofu Ceramiste Soft No. PA *(left)*; modified Shofu Ceramiste Soft No. PB *(right)*, which has a finer surface than PA.

Fig 8c Polishing completed before glazing.

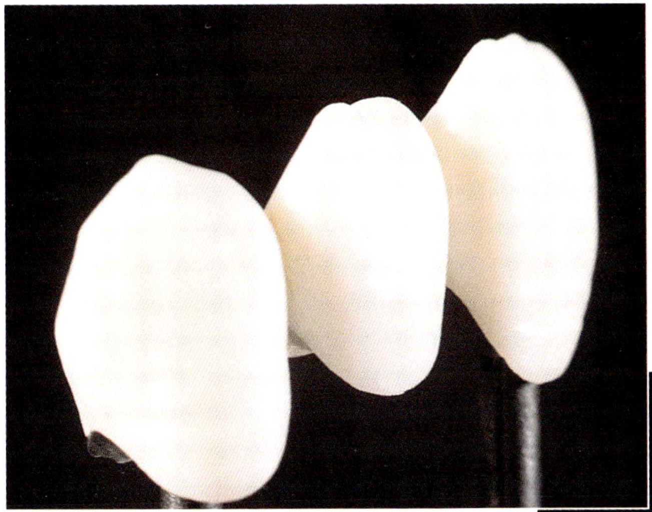

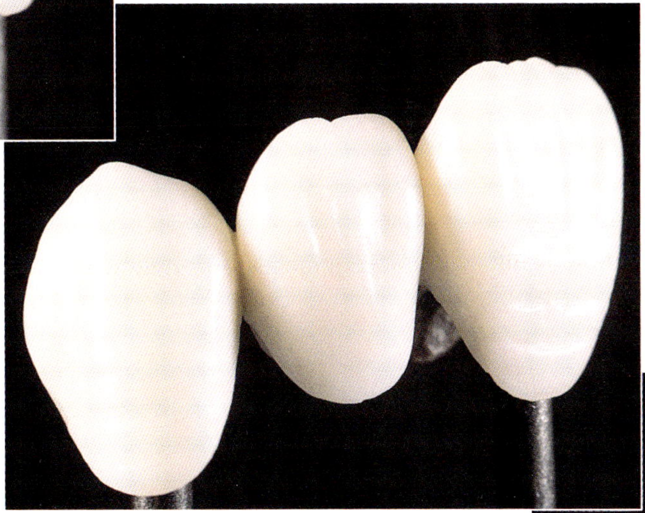

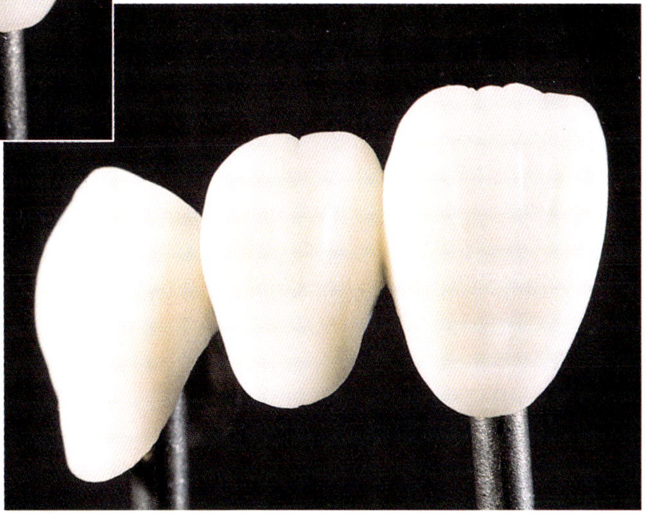

Fig 8d Fixed partial denture after glazing. Lateral view *(top)*; labial-lateral view *(middle)*; labial view *(bottom)*.

Emphasis

A modified Shofu Ceramiste Soft No. PA (Fig 8a) is used to polish the uneven surface of the porcelain. This modification allows the technician to follow the contours of the ridges and grooves. Likewise, a modified Shofu Ceramiste Soft No. PA or PB (Fig 8b) is used on the lingual side. Scratches are polished with these silicon points during contouring of surface characteristics, such as perikymata. After polishing, the fixed partial denture is glazed.

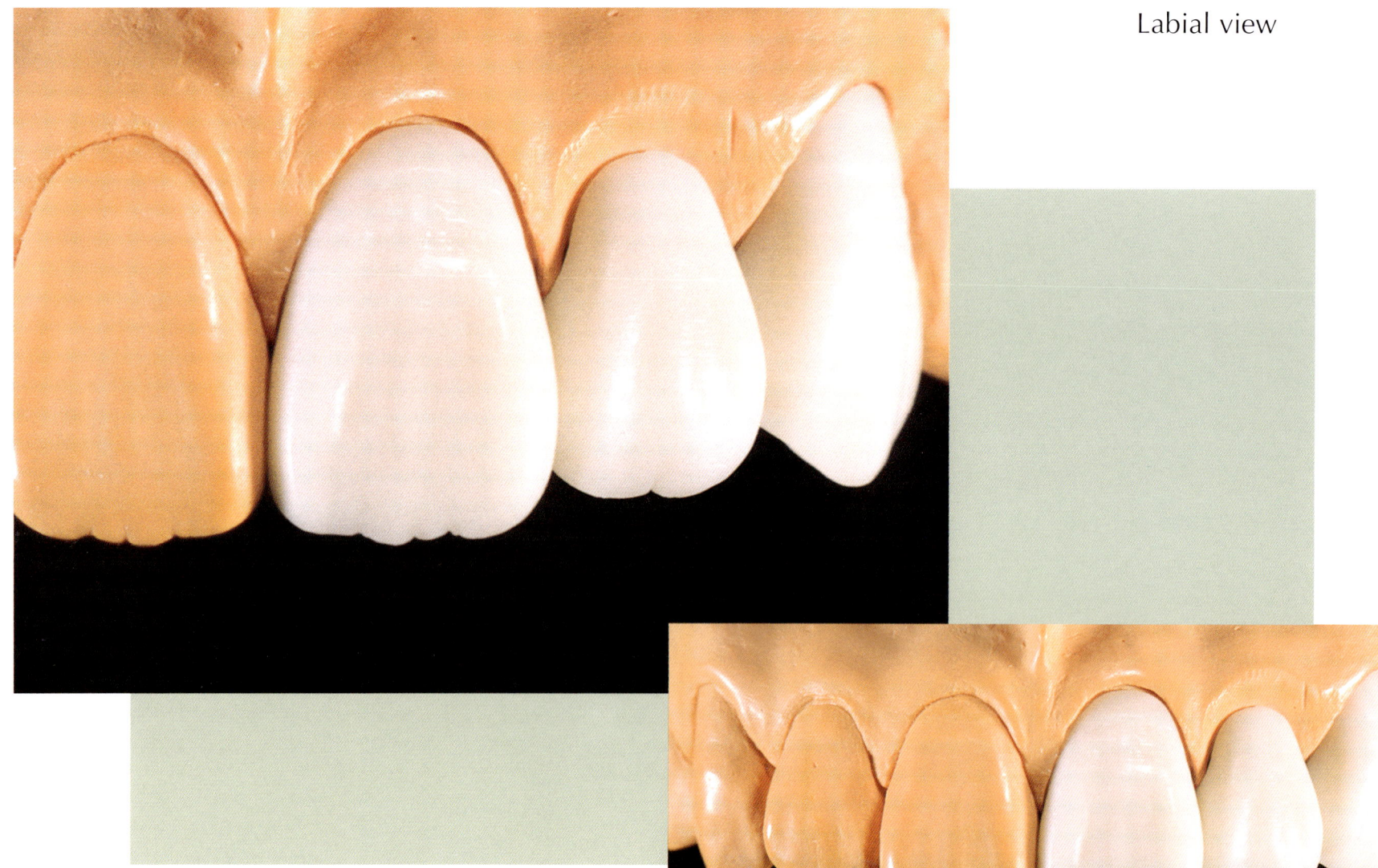

Completed Fixed Partial Denture

Labial view

Lingual view

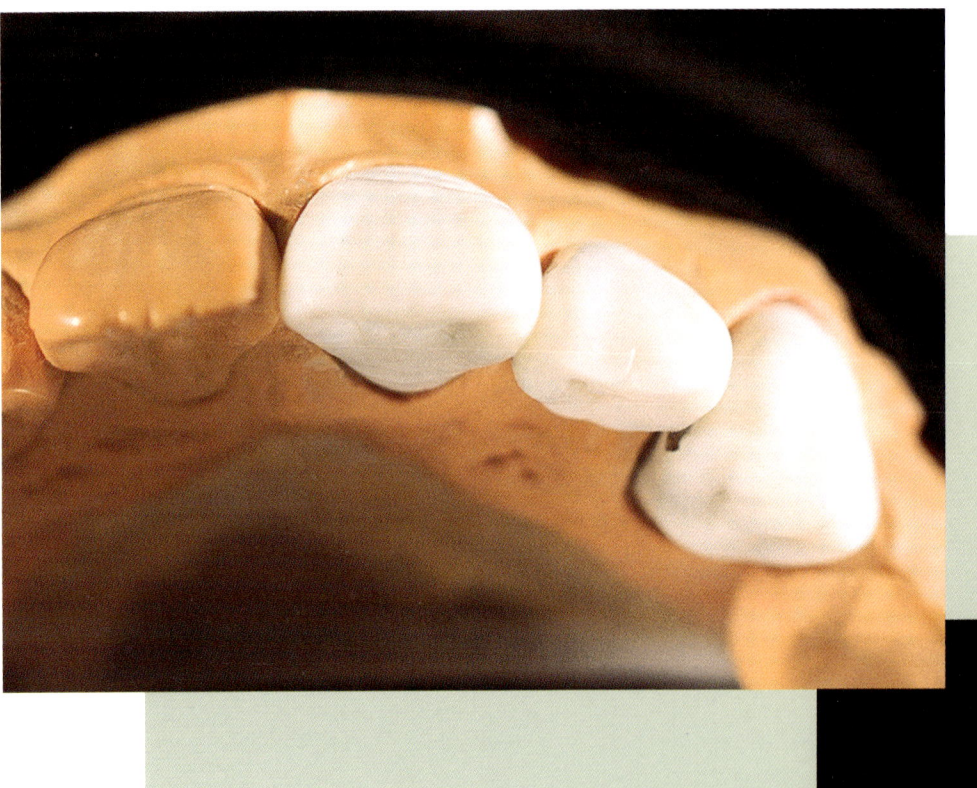

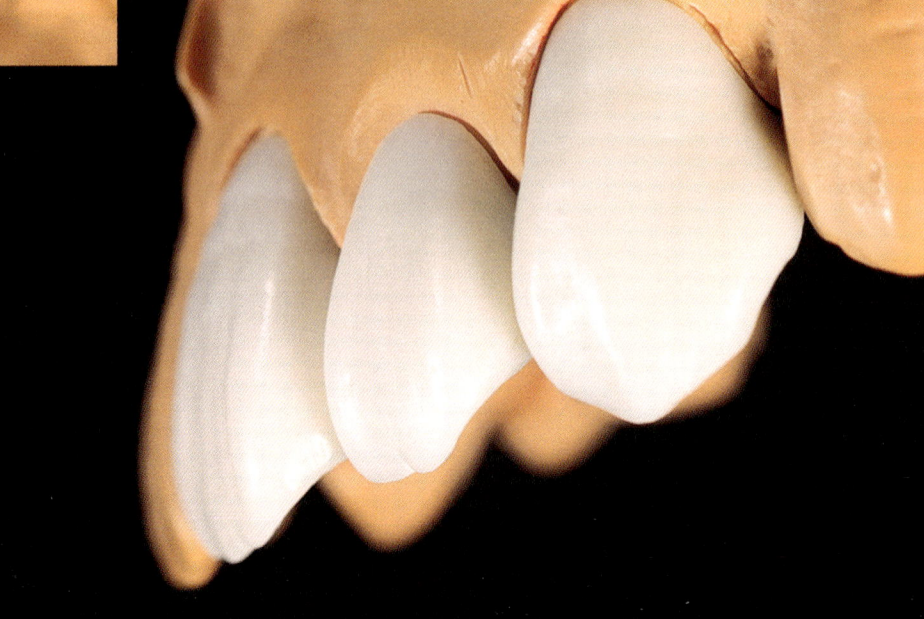

Completed Fixed Partial Denture

Incisal and lateral views